Meditation *and the* Meridians

Tian Li, L.Ac
and Norman Plotkin, CHt

Norman Plotkin Publishing
Fair Oaks, California, USA

Cover Design: Brittney Plotkin-Matone
Editing: Norman Plotkin, Brittney Plotkin-Matone

References: Wisdom without sickness by Qu Li Ming, TCM doctor, China

The Acupuncture Clinic Handbook by Jeffrey H. Jacob D.O.M, L.Ac

ISBN 978-1-7352354-3-1

Published 2023

TABLE OF CONTENTS

FOREWORD

This book was born of a project that we undertook in the tumultuous spring of 2020. After a new year vision of *having vision*, as in 20/20 vision, things got very complicated quickly. There were lockdowns and uncertainty. We just decided that we were not going to allow false evidence appearing real to cause us to lose our balance and harmony.

We expanded our individual meditation practices and in so doing expanded our peace of mind. We then decided, having seen efforts of others to spread love and calm through group meditations, to lead a weekly remote group meditation. Each Saturday night we would convene a group zoom meditation on various uplifting topics like love, gratitude and other related ideals.

After leading the meditations for a year we thought we might take the meditations in the direction of Traditional Chinese Medicine (TCM). Many meditation attendees learned about the meditations from the Tian Chao Herbs and Acupuncture community and were interested in a program that joined meditation and the meridians.

So, a sixteen week course on the meridians reinforced by meditations was developed and delivered. In the course a history and overview of TCM was shared and then the 12 main meridians were addressed, each with a commensurate meditation.

The pandemonium of the last several years has not happened outside of a larger context. We live in the time of a major epochal shift, the progression from one astrological age to another. Astrological ages follow a 2160-year cycle. According to John Fitzgerald in *The Astrological Journal*, the astrological ages are based on the precession of the equinoxes and the backwards wobble of the earth's axis through the constellations, which lie in a circle around the earth along the ecliptic belt of the equator.

Ages, Fitzgerald tells us, are measured by the wobble of the earth's axis and marks each age or constellation in succession. This wobble takes 25,920 years to complete, and in one complete cycle there are twelve ages (just like there are 12 main meridians!) of 2,160 years each. We are in the transition from the constellation Pisces, the *Age of Pisces* to the constellation Aquarius, the *Age of Aquarius*. These ages flow backward through the astrological signs as the earth's axis wobbles in a backward direction through the zodiac. This movement through the signs has a powerful influence on the history of each age.

The implications of this shift for earth and for humanity are tremendous and voluminous. The relevant aspects for this conversation are energetic. Remember, Qi is life force energy. And in the transition from Pisces to Aquarius we are experiencing a shift from material to energy, from Newtonian mechanics to the quantum field.

The distribution network called the meridian system looks like a giant web, linking different areas of our body together. Its pathways make up a comprehensive and complex body map that supplies vital *energy* to every part of the body.

Qi and meridians and energetic life force are terms that confuse Western medicine. Gross anatomy encompasses everything in the human body that is visible to the naked eye as well as areas that are visible through instrumental and surgical exploration and in cadavers through anatomical dissection.

A meridian is not an anatomical structure. Its morphology has not been in any way traced inside the human body. We are talking about a system of energy rather than material. Theories of TCM are constructed mainly upon the basis of philosophical thinking, emphasizing macro understanding of the body's functional status as a whole and thus rendering the anatomical description of human structures less important or even dispensable. Evidence based medicine describes Qi as a multipurpose principle having no analogue in modern scientific and biomedical terminology.

Qi is translated using expressions such as vital energy or vital life force. The part that confounds Western medicine is that dissection of a cadaver will never yield the meridians and you cannot order Qi from the pharmacy!

Meditation is part of the language of modern health. The practice has been around for millennia dating back thousands of years across many different cultures, and often shares elements with spirituality. Today, meditation is often used as an effective means of managing stress, anxiety, insomnia, and pain, among other chronic conditions. It can also be used to anchor new ideas and practices helping to create new neural pathways and overcome old ways of thinking or behaving.

Meditation lends itself well to helping people in this transition from material to energy. We found it to be an effective way to help open people's minds and hearts to understanding and embracing the world of meridians and Qi. We can never completely make our thoughts disappear; often, the more we try to suppress them, the louder they become. But practicing meditation can help clear away the mind's chatter.

Meditation is a mental exercise that trains attention and awareness. Its purpose is often to curb reactivity to one's negative thoughts and feelings, which, though they may be disturbing and upsetting and hijack attention from moment to moment, are invariably fleeting. Conversely, we can train our thoughts through meditation toward states that are desired.

When we understand that thoughts, especially negative ones, are fleeting, we can begin to release ourselves from the control they tend to have over us at times. And, through practice, we can train them toward desired realms.

The goal is to move into self-awareness. Self-awareness is your ability to perceive and understand the things that make you who you are as an individual, including your personality, actions, values, beliefs, emotions, and thoughts. Essentially, it is a psychological state in which the self becomes the focus of attention. And when we can train our self-awareness toward our mind, body and spirit, we are on our way to limitlessness.

Each chapter concludes with a meditation. You can record yourself reading the meditations and then play them back to yourself to achieve a guided meditative state. We hope you can find your way to limitlessness by understanding and applying meditation and the meridians!

Norman Plotkin
Sacramento, CA

INTRODUCTION

Meditation

According to *Psychology Today*, meditation is a mental exercise that trains attention and awareness. Its purpose is often to curb reactivity to one's negative thoughts and feelings, which, though they may be disturbing and upsetting and hijack attention from moment to moment, are invariably fleeting. When we understand that thoughts, especially negative ones, are fleeting, we can begin to release ourselves from the control they tend to have over us at times.

We can never completely make our thoughts disappear; often, the more we try to suppress them, the louder they become. But practicing meditation can help clear away the mind's chatter. Studies show that meditating even for as little as 10 minutes increases the brain's alpha waves (associated with relaxation) and decreases anxiety and depression.

The benefits of meditation are indisputable. Focus, concentration and balance are just a few of the positive aspects that come from meditation.

Health and healing begin in the mind, at the exact moment that we establish ourselves as in charge of our health. The first step in the health and healing processes, once decided and in charge, is to get control of your mind-talk, or self-talk.

All of your experiences, memories, and stored information stimulate the main activity of your mind and translate into self-talk. While we all collect negative experiences, we can also create capabilities for attention, concentration, mindfulness, and meditation. The challenge arises over the fact that we rarely use these capabilities because they require effort.

You express your self-talk through thoughts, images, sensations, and feelings, creating attitudes and behaviors that impact your daily life. Unhealthy self-talk leads to feelings of powerlessness as well as her step-sisters helplessness, inadequacy, and loneliness, which are experienced as isolation and deprivation.

These states are generally marked by self-talk that leads to emotional distress, anxiety, worry, and fear.

To promote healthy states of mind, we need to learn to take control of the predominantly automatic mental chatter that is self-talk; we need to take control by learning to practice mindfulness and learning meditation. Mindfulness and meditation are the first steps toward self-regulation and will allow us to find peace by relaxing our mind and body.

Meditation is a powerful tool to gain control of self-talk, which is the foundation for mindfulness, which in turn is the foundation of meditation and when accompanied by an understanding of and application to your meridian energy will lead to self-regulation and optimal health.

Meditation has been referred to as a fourth state by the Indian rishis, a state that is neither waking, nor sleeping, nor dreaming. And because it is outside normal experience, meditation will allow you to cut through all illusion, all projection, and all confusion you have about yourself and about others. But in order to reach this fourth state, your mind must transcend its normal activity.

Remember, all of your experiences, memories, and stored information stimulate the normal activity of your mind and translate into your self-talk. The problem is that this mind activity is influenced by perception and amplified by emotions.

You are always thinking, and most of the time you are experiencing emotions. But your thoughts don't mean anything; they are not who you are. Thoughts naturally come and go all of the time. In fact, it is estimated that we have as many as 60-70 thousand thoughts every day. It is further estimated that 90 percent of them are the same as the thoughts you had yesterday. When you attach yourself to your thoughts, you can and likely will, experience suffering.

Meditation is about coming face-to-face with your mind. Understand that this will lead you to penetrating insight into the illusions you have created in self-talk through the sometimes-distorted process of emotionally amplified perception.

Have you ever worked yourself to inaction when your overactive mind imagined every possible scenario and every possible negative outcome in a game of high speed, mental ping-pong?

People usually imagine that meditation is a technique that will train them to throw a psychological switch that will turn off the thinking and self-talk activity and leave the mind blank, calm, peaceful. That is not how it works.

Initially, thoughts, self-talk, and mental activity will continue. What changes is how you respond to them. Accept that thoughts will come. Greet them warmly and dismiss them without prejudice in a gentle exhale.

What follows is a written account of what originally appeared as a weekly meditation organized as a 13-part series on life mastery through bringing together meditation and the meridians of Traditional Chinese Medicine (TCM) into a focused program for balance, harmony and well-being. When our inner worlds and our outer worlds are balanced we can shape reality especially when we bring this balance into concerted action with others.

So, let's move from an overview of meditation to an introduction into the world of meridians.

Meridians

If you have been to see me in my clinic, Tian Chao Herbs and Acupuncture, or have seen another acupuncturist, you have no doubt heard about meridians.

The concept of meridians was derived merely from a very simple philosophical thinking: humans and nature bear resemblance to each other, the human body must therefore have a system of Qi and blood circulation similar to the flow of rivers and lakes in nature.

Ancient China was an agricultural society. Importantly, the condition of an irrigation system determined the harvest. And, as the way of human beings resembles that of heaven, the human body will certainly have a system of Qi and blood circulation similar to that of rivers and lakes in nature. The Yellow Emperor's Canon of Medicine has made it clear that as the Earth has four seas in the east, south, west and north, the human body must also have four "seas," namely, the sea of Shuigu (food digestion), the sea of Twelve Meridians, the sea of Qi and the sea of Marrow, and as there are twelve great rivers on earth, so there must be twelve meridians inside the human body.

Drawing analogy between the human body and nature is an evident feature of the philosophy of Traditional Chinese Medicine.

In TCM, there is a distribution network for the fundamental life force, Qi. Qi is a different concept from the common western understanding of the terms blood and bodily fluids. Qi is the foundation for maintaining health using Chinese medicine.

This distribution network called the Meridian System looks like a giant web, linking different areas of our body together. Its pathways make up a comprehensive and complex body map that supplies vital energy to every part of the body. Philosophically, the Meridian System explains how we live, and why we become sick.

Documents discovered in the Ma-Wang-Dui tomb in China, which was sealed in 198 BCE, contain no reference to acupuncture as such, but do refer to a system of meridians, albeit very different from the model that was accepted later. It is believed that the origin of meridians is closely related to the imageries derived by ancient physicians experiencing the circulation of Qi in their bodies during Qigong practice. As the renowned practitioner of the Ming dynasty, Li Shizhen, said in the Compendium of Materia Medica, "the interior channels of the body can only be detected by a self-observing person."

Jing-luo is the term in Chinese for the meridians, which are of extreme importance and serve as the cornerstone for understanding how the healing modalities in TCM operate. Jing Luo make up the basic structural components of the meridian system. These concepts can be traced back to China's oldest medical book The Yellow Emperor's Internal Classic from about 100 BC.

The Inner Classic information is presented in the form of questions by the Emperor and learned replies from his minister, Chi-Po. The text is likely to be a compilation of traditions handed down over centuries, presented in terms of the prevailing Taoist philosophy, and is still cited in support of particular therapeutic techniques.

The Inner Classic is divided into two parts, Su Wen and Ling Shu.

Su Wen addresses health and lifestyle maintenance. According to Su Wen, a long and healthy life awaits those who live in harmony with the seasons and conform to the rhythms of nature.

Lingshu generally discusses meridians and the circulation of Qi and blood.

In Chinese, Ling means the invisible and intangible spirit and soul. Shu means to pivot. Perhaps the spirit pivot is an esoteric way to describe the meridian as a transportation hub for metaphysical energetic flow.

Jing was originally an immovable silk thread drawn longitudinally from the loom. The jing of the meridian refers to the main path in the meridian system, which penetrates into the human body, penetrates up and down, and communicates inside and outside; Jing means pathway and refers to the vertical channels.

In Chinese, words can have multiple meanings based on tone and character variation. Luo, in this context, means collateral and refers to the auxiliary path branching out horizontally from the main path (jing), crisscrossing all over the body.

Both Jing and Luo mean link or connection. And they are bound closely together to form channels that TCM calls meridians.

Meridians are variably referred to as channels or collaterals based upon the difference in size and depth. There are twelve meridians, eight meridians of the odd meridian, and fifteen collaterals. The odd meridians, also referred to as the Eight Extraordinary Meridians represent the body's deepest level of energetic structuring. These meridians are the first to form in utero and are carriers of Yuan Qi, the ancestral energy which corresponds to our genetic inheritance. They function as deep reservoirs from which the twelve main meridians can be replenished, and into which the latter can drain their excesses.

We are going to focus on the twelve-meridian system. The twelve meridians resemble a river, and the circulation is endless; the odd meridian is like a lake, quiet and deep, hidden; the twelve meridians are the internal communication apparatus of the human body, which originate from the ends of the limbs and connect the internal organs. And the eight channels of the odd meridian are storage of the essence. The twelve meridians and the eight odd meridians are connected by collaterals.

Qi and meridians and energetic life force are terms that confound Western, or allopathic medicine. Gross anatomy is the historical and factual basis of scientific medicine. It encompasses everything in the human body that is visible to the naked cye as well as areas that are visible through instrumental and surgical exploration and in cadavers through anatomical dissection; that is to say, gross anatomy includes all organs, structures, and portions thereof.

A meridian is not an anatomical structure. Its morphology has not been in any way traced inside the human body. Even more importantly, theories of TCM are constructed mainly upon the basis of philosophical thinking, emphasizing macro understanding of the body's functional status as a whole and thus rendering the anatomical description of human structures less important or even dispensable.

The meridian theory has apparently reflected the perceptual characteristics of Chinese culture for its direct image visualization with intuitive logic, which must be a key point when we discuss the origin of meridians.

According to a review by evidence based medicine, Qi is a multipurpose principle having no analogue in modern scientific and biomedical terminology; the term is translated using expressions such as vital energy or vital life force.

The irony is that dissection of a cadaver will not yield the meridians and you cannot order Qi from the pharmacy!

Does that mean it does not exist? Herein lies the philosophical versus physiological debate between Western Medicine and TCM. And this question could involve a whole paper unto itself. But as we move past the materialism of Newtonian mechanics and into the quantum field, energy medicine and energy healing is becoming more widely accepted and understood.

TCM is considered a mystical science by some skeptics. However, nothing about it is mysterious once you grasp its underlying concepts. TCM draws on Taoist philosophy that is rooted in the laws and synergies of nature, and it applies these synergies to the human body. It recognizes that our organ systems are interconnected and our health is dependent on chi. Translated to modern-day language, chi is active energy, a metaphor for metabolic processes taking place in a living being. To be alive is to have vital chi flowing through the body.

While in this framework the body is understood as a harmonious and coherent totality of a variety of physiological systems, the meridians are the channels that give unity to the whole.

It is precisely through these linking points that the Qi becomes more readily accessible and it is on them that acupuncture practitioners operate to manipulate the flux of Qi by employing a variety of techniques including the use of needles, finger pressure, cupping, and so on.

What makes such interventions therapeutically important is that according to the existing theories about etiology and pathogenesis in TCM, disease arises when an imbalance exists between the different energies of the human body through Qi excess or deficiency or alternatively when an excess of air, dryness, heat, or cold occurs either due to the influence of the environment or for entirely internal reasons.

In terms of Western medicine, in the face of a given organic condition, manipulating the meridians leads to a correction of such forms of imbalance and thus the restoration of health.

But Western materialism will never be satisfied of the scientific foundation of a therapeutic framework that by its own admission has at its very foundation a recognition of the undetectability of Qi. Therefore, Qi and the river of meridians through which it flows will be forever philosophical rather than physiological in nature.

So while we are considering Qi and meridians philosophically, it might help to think of these acupuncture meridians as streams or rivers flowing with energy or information. Like a river that provides water to its surrounding areas, these channels distribute energy and carry information to the surrounding area of the body. The body can then carry out the instructions.

Since Qi and blood are mobile, it's easier to understand the concept of meridian by comparing it to water flow, just as the ancients who conceived of the concept did. When water flows down a mountain or a slope, it flows from a high to low ground and will also follow the geographical terrain and collect in the most stable area which is a river. Rivers maintain the natural laminar, or smooth, flow, providing the most efficient way of transporting water downstream. As a result, the land surrounding the river is lush with vegetation and life because of the steady supply of fresh water.

Qi works in a similar way to the flow of water in nature. By flowing from a high to low concentration, it follows the body's landscape and gathers in a meridian. Thus, meridians provide a natural pathway for the flow of Qi and supply a constant source of energy to different parts of the body in the same way a river supplies water to its surrounding banks.

If a river is blocked, all areas relying on the water downstream will be affected. Due to a lack of water, the ecosystem's balance and harmony are disturbed. And plants and animals cannot survive. Similarly, if the meridian system is blocked, the supply of Qi to different parts of the body will be interrupted. Leading to organ disharmony and disease even if the affected area is far away from the original blockage.

Meridians work like a network system, transporting and distributing Qi and blood. They link up organs, limbs, joints, bones, tendons, tissues and skin, and provide communication between the body interior and exterior, through a healthy meridian system. Qi and blood successfully warm and nourish different organs and tissues, and maintain normal metabolic activities. Meridians are essential in supporting the flow of nutritive Qi inside the blood vessels and flow of protective Qi around them. In addition, they strengthen the body's immunity, protect against external pernicious influences and assist in regulating Yin and Yang.

The beginning of any disease can be traced back to the disturbance of life energy, not the destruction of the material organs. Any destruction is an accumulation process. When it accumulates to a certain extent, it comes on like a landslide. Therefore, everyone must pay attention to this initial energy interference. This energy interference refers to the inhibition or obstruction of life caused by the five elements, or pain caused by the obstruction of the meridians. If we look at the disease in a purely material way, it can only mean that the disease has taken shape, and it is difficult to treat. When the disease is not taking shape, the imbalance of energy can be adjusted and it can be cured. This is the essential meaning of preventive medicine to life.

The best doctor is yourself; the best medicine is your meridians.

"Lingshu·Meridian" says: "The meridian, therefore, can resolve all diseases, treat all kinds of diseases, and regulate the deficiency and excess." It means that the smoothness of the meridian system is related to the body's disease, life and death.

Because of the special properties of meridians and their correlation to imbalance in the body, conditions can be diagnosed according to the meridian and its corresponding organ. Headaches, for example, are classified according to their affected painful spots and the distribution of the meridians in that area.

Two areas of life energy affect the twelve meridians. First, emotions, such as love and hate, fear and pride, are all energy that fluctuates at any time in daily life. When emotions fluctuate, such as stress or anger, the meridians are immediately blocked, and then the organs, the stomach, and the liver are injured. Long-term resentment also hurts the lungs, the heart, and the liver. Happiness can keep you in good health, because happiness opens meridians.

Next is the environment. Good and bad environments also affect life energy. Good mountains and good waters are definitely beneficial to life. This is not just about the living environment and feng shui. The larger environment is the stage of life you are in. Everyone can achieve life goals and inspiration. In a good stage of life filled with motivation, the perceived value of one's life will be more meaningful and healthier.

What is the importance of learning the meridian system?

Assuming that our body is a house that needs to be refurbished, what should we do before refurbishing this house?

First of all, we need to understand the structure of the house. Using this analogy, we must first understand the structure of the human body's internal organs, the distribution of the eight channels of odd meridians, and the direction of the 12 meridians and the circulation of Qi and blood.

For example, the meridians of the face, with the nose as the center, mainly go through the stomach meridian, so the thick pores on both sides of the nose are related to the lack of stomach Qi, and daily massage of Zhongwan acupoint is a good way to fill the stomach with Qi. Zhongwan Point is four inches above the belly button. Although it belongs to the Ren Channel, it is also the recruiting point of the Foot Yangming Stomach Meridian. Recruiting means gathering, so Zhongwan Point is the gathering of Qi in the Foot Yangming Stomach Meridian.

After we progress through this course about the twelve meridians, we will know that there are several large parts of the human body that are very important, such as the Empty basin (Stomach 12 - Que Pen), such as the underarms, such as the Qi Street at the base of the thigh, where the meridians gather.

What are these important points? Maintenance. For the Empty basin, we can put the Palace of labor (Pericardium 8 - Laogong) acupoint on the right hand on the left shoulder and cover the Empty Basin every day when we sleep. The armpits need to be rubbed. Three of the acupuncture points are beneficial to the armpits: one is the Celestial Gathering (Small Intestine 11 -Tianzong) acupoint on the shoulder blade, the other is the Great Embrace (Spleen 21 - Dabao) acupoint below the armpit, and the other is the Highest Spring (Heart 1 - Jiquan) acupoint under the armpit.

For many women, these three acupuncture points are particularly painful when rubbed. This is the year-round depression of qi and blood stasis. After rubbing it, it will be fine. The Qijie acupoint at the base of the thigh needs to be slapped, which is good for gynecology as well as men's prostate. For these three points, you have to spend 15 minutes every day. So, meridian health care takes effort, but this effort is spent on raising one's health. Put down the phone for 15 minutes, do eye exercises, pat the thighs, and close your eyes.

By connecting and uniting different parts of our body, meridians provide the transport service for the fundamental substances of Qi, blood, and body fluids. The flow of Qi in the Meridian System concentrates or "injects" in certain areas of the skin's surface. These areas are very small points known as acupuncture points. Although acupuncture points are located externally and superficially, they can affect the internal functions of our body. There are 365 acupuncture points, and each point belongs to a particular meridian channel that connects to specific organs.

Classification of Meridians

The Meridian System has 12 principal meridians that correspond to the Yin and Yang organs and the pericardium. Yin organs are usually those without an empty cavity, and include the liver, heart, spleen, lungs, and kidneys. Yang organs are organs with an empty cavity such as the gallbladder, small intestine, stomach, large intestine and bladder.

In TCM, Yin and Yang organs are physiologically functional units that incorporate a much broader meaning than traditional western thinking. Logically, meridians linked with Yin organs are known as Yin meridians; if they are linked to Yang organs, they are known as Yang meridians. As noted above, in addition to the12 principal meridians, there are eight extra meridians also known as odd meridians. Among the eight extra meridians, the Du meridian (Governing Vessel) and Ren meridian (the Conception Vessel) are considered the most important channels, because they contain acupuncture points which are independent of the twelve principal meridians.

The twelve regular meridians are distributed symmetrically on both sides of the body, are paired with their corresponding internal organs and have lateral and symmetrical distribution on the head, face, trunk and limbs. The 6 Yin meridians are distributed on the inner side of the limbs, and on the chest and abdomen. The 6 Yang meridians are distributed on the outer side of the limbs and on the head, face, trunk and back.

The order and arrangement of the 12 regular meridians result in particular ways of communication inside the body. TCM uses Yin/Yang characteristics to distinguish and understand the patterns of meridian flow.

The daily Qi current divides among the 12 meridians over 12 two hour periods.

Arm: Lung Meridian: 3 am - 5 am, Large intestine: 5 am - 7 am
Leg: Stomach Meridian: 7 am - 9 am, Spleen Meridian: 9 am - 11 am
Arm: Heart Meridian: 11 am - 1pm, Small intestine: 1 pm - 3 pm
Leg: Bladder Meridian: 3 pm - 5pm, Kidney Meridian: 5 pm - 7pm
Arm: Pericardium Meridian: 7 pm - 9 pm, Triple Warmer: 9 pm - 11 pm
Leg: Gallbladder: 11 pm – 1 am, Liver: 1 am - 3 am.

In the following chapters we will dive into each of the main meridians, each meridians' particular characteristics, associated organs and emotions.

As shown above, Qi is more prevalent in different meridians at different times. For example, from 3 am to 5 am, meridian Qi mainly flows through the lung meridian, if people wake up that time, or cough, or wake up with a headache etc., that means lung energy is off or stressed. Then the Qi enters the large intestine meridian at 5 am - 7 am, if you wake up by abdomen cramp and need to move your bowel then that means you have healthy large intestine. And then the stomach meridian from 7 am – 9 am, it's the best time to have breakfast. I have always told people to finish your breakfast before 9 am. It's the best way to take care of your digestion. In this way, the meridian cycle is continuous as the Qi flows through the body.

The meridians start in the lung meridian and end in the liver meridian. The birth of a person begins with the activation of lung Qi, crying; it also ends with the extinction of liver Qi and let go.

At the end of each meridian chapter there will be an addendum in which we build a meditation around these properties to enhance balance, health and well-being associated with each of the individual meridians.

Meridians Meditation

Resting comfortably now.

Feeling safe, calm, and at ease.

I want you, to give yourself permission, to take this time, just for you.

I want you to relax, and just for a little while at least, I want you to let go.

Let go of all the thoughts of responsibility that would normally preoccupy your mind.

But for now, there is nothing at all to stop you from taking this time to just relax - to relax, and enjoy the feeling of returning to your natural state of simply just being.

So allowing your eyes, to softly close now…

Send the thought of relaxation all the way down to your toes… just let your toes relax…

Now allow that relaxation to move up your body… up your spine… across your shoulders… up to the top of your head…

I want you to experience now, a beautiful violet stream of light, pouring down from the sky like a laser beam, in through the crown of your head.

The violet light symbolizes purity of thought, as now you experience only positive thoughts and feelings, as far as is humanly possible.

And the purity of thought and feeling touches every meridian and acupoint - filling you with a new healthy Qi, a strong and positive life-force energy - and you feel yourself filled with a loving acceptance of yourself.

Your feelings are changing on a cellular level… feel the chemistry of your body being altered in a positive way… fortifying your meridians and balancing your Qi.

You can just allow yourself, to feel free.

Free to relax, and enjoy the feeling, of having nothing at all, to bother your mind.

Nothing at all, to think about.

Nothing, other than, the here, and now. There is no time but now, there is no place but here.

And right here, and now - all you need to focus on is the air that you breathe.

Breathe in a universal energy that is your life force, your Qi.

So breathing deeply, and easily now.

Now, just let your mind go now, let it wander just as it will.

Pause…

Only aware of your thoughts and my voice now.

Now… it is time to expand our sacred journey of transformation…

Take a deep and cleansing breath.

Let's simply bring your awareness to the breath

Take a deep breath… inhale and exhale…

In this moment, this here and now, you are powerful and you are confident and you can transform yourself… let a deep sensation of confident calm flow throughout your body now… throughout the extensive system of your meridians and the river system of your life-force, qi…let the sensation lift all that it touches…

Breathing in relaxation, exhaling any tension or stress…

As we move through this meditative journey, let's pause a moment and allow ourselves to fully be… here, present, now…

Pause…

Return to the sound of my voice… and allow the energy of my voice to take you deeper into relaxation as we begin an imagery journey…

Allow your shoulders to drop and relax, and plant your feet firmly on the ground... Or, if you are sitting cross-legged, feel the sense of contact between your feet and the seat and the floor beneath you.

Quell your analytical mind if need be with the understanding that Qi is a multipurpose principle having no analogue in modern scientific and biomedical terminology… understand that the term Qi is translated using expressions such as vital energy or vital life force.

Accept that dissection of a cadaver will never yield the meridians and you cannot order qi from the pharmacy… but rather it is the product of subtle intuitive logic formed from the observations of nature herself…

Know that Qi works in a similar way to the flow of water in nature ... By flowing from a high to low concentration, it follows the body's landscape and gathers in a meridian… Thus, meridians provide a natural pathway for the flow of Qi and supply a constant source of energy to different parts of the body in the same way a river supplies water to its surrounding banks...

Understand that if a river is blocked, all areas relying on the water downstream will be affected ... lack of water translates to the ecosystem's balance and harmony being disturbed...

Similarly, if the meridian system is blocked, the supply of Qi to different parts of the body will be interrupted.... organ disharmony and disease follow even if the affected area is far away from the original blockage...

Pause…

Now for the next few breaths bring your full focus of attention to your breathing.

Notice the feeling of the air flowing in through the nostrils, down into the lungs, and down into the belly as you inhale...

And on the exhale, feel the release of any tension as you let the air out slowly ...

I want you to go back in your mind now - back through time.

Go back in time, further and further back through your teens, your childhood. Just let your mind wander gently back in time, as though there is no such thing as time.

Pause...

Let your mind travel back now - and see yourself, becoming smaller, and younger, younger and smaller.

You may feel as though you are swirling through a long tunnel or mist - or travelling over the bridge of time.

Pause...

Good, now see yourself as though you are watching a screen with a movie being shown on it.

Continuing to breathe, deeply, and easily, now, allowing yourself, to let go, let go, and relax. Let yourself travel back in time.

Let go, of all the strain, and all the tension of present moments, simply allowing it, to evaporate, and disappear, becoming more and more relaxed.

Let go, of anything that no longer serves you - and watch, as it floats upwards, and drifts away.

Leaving you feeling calmer - calmer and more relaxed.

Much calmer, and much, much, more relaxed, with each, and every breath, you take.

Feeling more peaceful, and completely - awash, with pure relaxation.

You are possibly starting to feel so relaxed, by now. As you travel all the way back into your mother's womb.

Pause...

See yourself forming in vitro. The branches of your meridians being formed…

First your collateral meridians, those that carry your ancestral information… deep and wide… filling with qi, the reservoirs that will hold your Qi to replenish your Jing-luo.

Only aware of your thoughts and my voice now ... as the scene unfolds in your mind…

The pathways of your main meridians being laid down now, your river system for life-force energy…

Become aware of the importance of this formation… become aware of this life-force energy… understand that managing the balance of this system will lead to health, wellness and longevity…

Pause…

I want the adult you, who is here now listening to me, to go back and visit that developing meridian system.

See yourself as you are now, discovering that system.

Quickly make friends with your life-force qi and your meridian system.

Vow to nurture this system… vow to act in ways that are in harmony with the flow of life… the change of seasons… pledge to yourself that you will always be aware of the impact of your environment and your emotions on your qi and its river system of meridians…

Pause…

The more you listen to your meridians, the more you learn and understand.

And if anything should start to bother you again in the future, whether it's your body, pain, discomfort, you know that you can go back inside and get in touch with your meridians to find out exactly what the problem or problems might be....

You now know that you can, like a Qi Gong master, pinpoint and correct whatever it is that's causing you concern, and with the help and guidance of your meridians once again your life will become stress free and a most wonderful and enjoyable experience.

Pause…

Now what may happen in the future is that sometimes you just get that feeling that you want to go inside for a short while and revisit your life-force system and although consciously you may not be aware that you are with it, the deeper part of your mind becomes reconciled to a feeling of total unity within you, and this creates a beneficial sensation of harmony and inner peace.

Pause…

You notice that you feel differently about any and all negative feelings and emotions which may have been troubling you, sensing that from now on everything's going to be fine, it will all work out for the best as your unconscious mind continues to protect you in a way that allows you to be healthy, energetic and balanced…

Pause…

When you return in a few moments to the here and now after this session bring back with you new insights - new learning's, new possibilities and new avenues for you to explore.

Pause…

Now that you have come through this meditation, notice how you feel in your body… how happy you feel… Take a moment to take three slow, deep breaths and feel how wonderful it is to live a life filled with happiness…

Now just breathe and be present with yourself for a moment, and then come back when you are ready…

CHAPTER ONE

Lung Meridian

Characteristics

The lung meridian is called the "Prime Minister" and assists with controlling energy and circulating the blood. The lungs and the heart are seen to work in conjunction with blood and energy, being complementary parts of the living system. This connection has led the lungs to also be called "The Priest" and the "Minister of Heaven." The lungs also control the skin and perspiration.

This meridian generates what is known as the radiant energy. This control puts the lungs in the front line for fighting external disease.

The meridians start in the lung meridian and end in the liver meridian. The birth of a person begins with the activation of lung Qi, crying; it also ends with the extinction of liver Qi and let go.

From three am to five am, meridian Qi mainly flows through the lung meridian. If people wake up at that time, or cough, or wake up with a headache, etc., that means lung energy is off or stressed; and then enters the large intestine Meridian at five am to seven am. If you wake up with an abdomen cramp and need have a bowel movement, this means you have a healthy large intestine.

If not, then work on your large intestine meridian. And then the stomach meridian from seven am to nine am. This the best time to have breakfast, I have always told my patients to finish their breakfast before nine am. It's the best way to take care of your digestion. In this way, the meridian cycle is continuous as the Qi flows through the body.

Lung Meridian

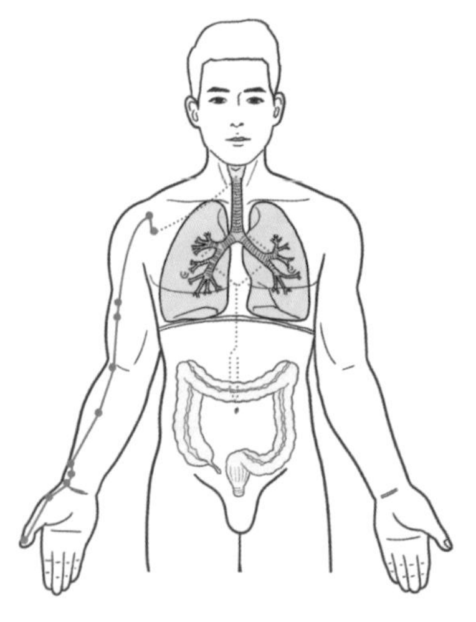

Primary Pathway

The Lung Meridian primary pathway originates in the middle portion of the body, and runs downward connecting with the large intestine. It then turns and passes through the diaphragm to connect with the lungs. This meridian branches out from the axilla (armpit) and runs down the medial aspect of the upper arm where it crosses the elbow crease.

It continues until it passes above the major artery of the wrist, and emerges at the tip of the thumb. Another branch emerges from the back of the wrist and ends at the radial side of the tip of the index finger to connect with the Large Intestine Meridian.

Characteristics of lungs

The lungs are dedicated organs. The lung is the weakest organ in our body. The lung is the first organ that a baby needs to activate after coming out of the mother's womb. The first thing a child must do as it is being born from the mother is to open the lobes of the lungs. Crying is used to open the lobes of the lung. What does the doctor or midwife do if the baby doesn't cry at this time? A swift pat to the buttocks and then the soles of the feet.

The lung, located as the top source of five organs, is the first organ to feel the harm of the environment and the first organ to be affected by medications. If kids catch a cold or flu or eat the wrong foods, drink some ginger soup and massage the belly. It will be ok. I'm most afraid that the parents will rush to eliminate the symptoms and mess up the child's blood and energy. Life has to be slowly transformed, and time must be given to the movement of Qi and blood. Usually, it is best to let the children get more sun, exercise more, and eat less sweets, so that the lungs can be strong.

As we know, the lung is in charge of breathing. The best breathing is what is often referred to as belly breathing, or breathing deeply down to the lower Dantian, which is in the area a few fingers below your navel. This type of breathing involves the kidney's energy, so chronic respiratory system problems actually require work on the lung and kidney too. The best breathing exercise is Qi Gong breathing exercises.

The lungs are in charge of dispersing and descending. After the meridian Qi returns to the lungs, the lungs will also distribute the twelve meridian Qi to the whole body. This kind of redistribution is strict, and it's not something any organ can have more than others.

If the lung Qi is not descending, the quality of people's sleep will be poor. The time for the lungs to distribute energy is from three to five am, so sleeping deeply at this time is important.

The lungs are also in charge of the skin and hair. Skin diseases like eczema, psoriasis, etc., are primarily associated with the lungs. Skin diseases originate at the joints, which is characteristic of lung disease. The second characteristic is symmetry because the meridians are symmetric. For example, the most common eczema flare place is at He Gu (large intestine 4) area.

Lungs are deeply affected by grief, sadness and worry. People with severe skin problems almost universally also have grief, sadness and worry too. So, it doesn't matter how much topical medicine you put on skin, if the lung meridian has not been addressed, and the emotion has never been recognized and dealt with, the skin problem will never go away.

The lungs are partnered with the large intestine, they are in the same family, so to speak. These two meridians also share the same tissue in western medicine. If lung cancer ranks first, then large intestine cancer will be second.

TCM Lung organ

It is important to remember that the lung organ in Chinese medicine is not the lung organ referred to by western medicine. The TCM lung organ is like a system, it also includes the lung meridians, including the relationship between the lung and the body, and the relationship between the lung and the skin. Even if the lung lobes are removed, the relationship between the lung meridian and other meridians is still there, and it will work.

Main Indication

Acupuncture points in the Lung Meridian are indicated for throat, chest and lung ailments and for other symptoms that are presented along the meridian's pathway. Imbalances in the lung meridian can cause upper respiratory infection, breathing dysfunction, and skin problems. An imbalance can also cause despair and depression.

Symptoms

Disorders of the Lung Meridian lead to diseases related to TCM lung dysfunction. According to TCM, the lung rules and regulates Qi throughout the body and administers respiration (breathing). In addition, the lung moves and adjusts the water channels, so disorders of this meridian may be related to disharmony of lung fluid or "water" and respiratory disorders. Symptoms like chest discomfort with a fullness sensation, dyspnea (shortness of breath), cough, and wheezing indicate Lung Meridian disharmony. This disharmony can also lead to pain along the meridian position.

Examples include, but are not limited to, pain or cold feeling in the upper arms, indicating weak heart and lungs; blue veins that pop out on the lateral tail of the elbow indicating that the lungs are cold and allergic; The thenar (known as the big fish area) should be a nice pink color, if it is blueish, wrinkly, or pale it means the lung is cold; and cold stomach too.

Deficiency of lung Qi

Signs of lung Qi deficiency include weak urination. Irregular stool is another indication including weak and incomplete stool and soft stool. By contrast, babies who have enough lung Qi have quick bowel movements that are firm and thick.

Other signs of lung Qi deficiency include cold and pain in the upper arms and shoulder and frequent sighs or shortness of breath.

Healthy Lung

Deep sleep between three and five am is a sign of a healthy lung meridian. Interrupted sleep at this time points to lung Qi deficiency.

The phrase "cold injures the lungs" explains the root of lung disease. In this day and age, people don't pay enough attention to keeping warm when they are young, and drink too many iced beverages. Not only can these behaviors cause allergies, they can also injure internal organs and result in coughs. And chronic pharyngitis is often caused by taking the wrong or too many medications.

It is super important to develop a good, mindful lifestyle. Wear boots, hats and a scarf in fall and winter, don't wear sandals and flip flops. And don't sweat profusely in the summer. Don't eat food that is too cold or too hot. Too much cold food and cold drinks particularly hurt the lungs. And don't sleep too late.

The best way to protect the delicate lungs is to protect them from cold. Consume fewer or no cold drinks and foods. The best exercise is swimming. In addition, do deep breathing QI Gong and engage in lung meridian massage. Take all medications with caution. And finally and of utmost importance, manage your emotions, Grief, sadness and worry can hurt the lungs. The first step to bring lung health back is to manage our emotions.

Acupoints

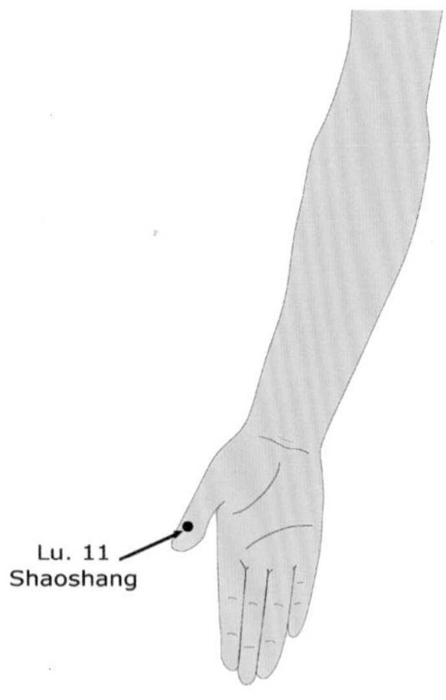

LU 11: SHAO SHANG (LESSER METAL)

Name: Lesser Metal, Shang is the sound of metal. Gathers Da Qi, great Qi.
Location: the corner of the big thumb nail, at the radial (lateral) aspect of the thumb.
Indication: Asthma, sore throat, cough, nose bleeding, high fever.
Techniques and notes: massage or prick the point to cause bleeding.
This point is particularly good for emergency situations like fever, sore throat, and tonsillitis. You can use a lancet needle to prick LU11, and squeeze 5-10 drops of black blood, throat immediately less painful; fever can drop right away; you can also bleed from the tip of the ear too, which is also an effective way for high fever.

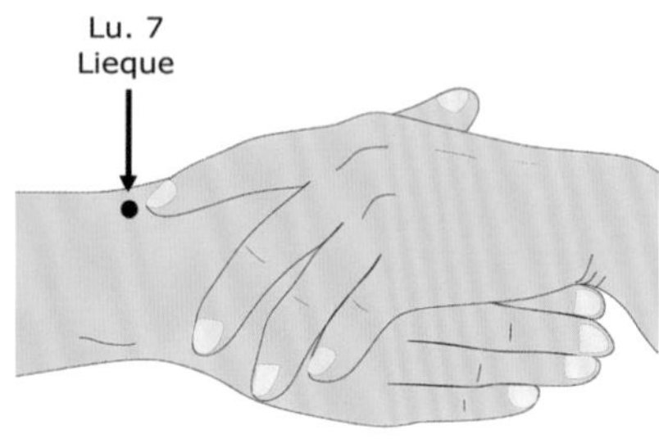

LU 7: LIE QUE (BROKEN SEQUENCE)

Name: Broken Sequence, is the god of thunder and lightning, connecting up and down.
Location: to find Lie que: cross the fingers with the left and right hands, and press the index finger of one hand on the styloid process of the other hand. There is a small hollow, which is the Lie que point.
Indications: Flu, common cold, headache, asthma, sore throat, toothache, facial paralysis.
Techniques and notes: massage. For help trigeminal neuralgia, memory loss. Massage 1-3 mins every day.

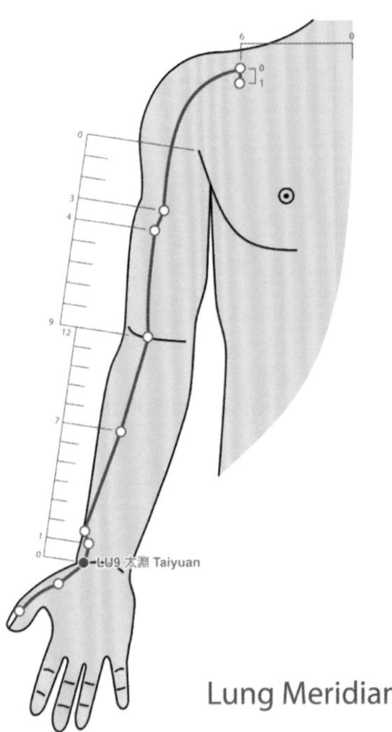

Lung Meridian

LU 9: TAI YUAN (GREAT ABYSS)

Name: Great Abyss, an abyss that is the source of water. Tai Yuan can connect the twelve meridians, all the collaterals meet here, it is their meeting place.

Location: Taiyuan is located on the wrist, with the palm up, on the first horizontal line behind the palm, touching the place where the pulse is pulsed.

Indications: Cough, cold, asthma, chest pain, fainting, low energy, depression, skin issue, local pain. It's a good curative effect on blood disorders and blood circulation diseases. Very good for high blood pressure.

Techniques and notes: First thing every morning, rub the Taiyuan acupoint for a few minutes, which can continuously transport vitality for the circulating source Qi, and can ensure the energy and vitality for the heart. When you have shortness of breath, or asthma massaging it for four to five minutes can relieve the symptoms.

Miscellaneous bits

Official: Prime Minister
Sense Organ: Nose
Body Fluid: Nasal Discharge
Element: Metal
Direction: West
Season: Autumn
Climate: Dry
Sense: Smell

Tissue: Skin and Hair
Positive Emotion: Courage
Negative Emotion: Grief, Sadness
Spiritual: Po- Corporeal Soul
Flavor: Pungent (Umami)
Color: White
Sound: Crying
Time: 3 am to 5 am
Origin/Ending: Mid stomach to Hand
Number of Acupoints: 11 on each side, total 22 on both sides of the body.

Lung Meditation

When you are comfortable, I would like you to gently close your eyes and focus your attention onto the sound of my voice.

As you listen now, I would like you to become aware of your body and how your clothes feel against your skin.

Can you imagine feeling completely relaxed? I wonder if you could take a nice deep breath in, and as you release the breath slowly, let go of all the tension in those muscles around your body.

You already know how to breathe deeply so allow yourself to enjoy all the sensations of a deep breath in and breathing out all the tensions as you relax.

Short pause.

Let's go on a sacred meditative journey of transformation…

Returning now to your breath, you know that each gentle out-breath can lead to more and more relaxation.

Paying attention to your breathing can help you relax even more.

This is your own special time that you have set aside just for you, because you don't need to be anywhere or do anything apart from concentrate on your breathing and relax all those muscles.

There is no time, but now, there is no place but here and right now and right here, you are safe, supported and relaxed.

On a subtle level you understand… all the parts of your body are made of molecules, atoms and sub-atomic particles, and these are in constant motion… Try to really get a feeling for the change that is taking place each moment in your body…. This will help you begin to understand Qi…

Feel how your awareness of your meridians empowers you to alter your body's balance; how your meridian awareness can provide the opportunity to not only shift from wherever you are to balance and harmony, but also to project love and kindness to others…

Embrace the fact that over the course of 2,500 years, Traditional Chinese Medicine has become a tried and tested system of rational medicine known for its great diversity of healing and wellness practices ... know that the main goal of TCM is to create harmony between our mind, body, and the environment around us...

Know that oftentimes, physical symptoms can be made worse by, or even result from, an imbalance of energy in your body rather than an issue in the particular spot where you are experiencing discomfort ... understand that health is all about balance, and when it is thrown off, you become more susceptible to disease ... Energy is the director of your body's harmony; its movement is crucial to your health...

Understand too that one very important way to create harmony is by making sure your Qi is balanced ... Qi means life energy and it stands for the energy in all things...

Embrace the opportunity to nurture your lung meridian… know that the lung meridian is known as the "Prime Minister" and assists with controlling energy and circulating the blood. Understand that the lungs and the heart are seen to work in conjunction with blood and energy, being complementary parts of the living system… This connection has led the lungs to also be called "The Priest" and the "Minister of Heaven." The lungs also control the skin and perspiration…

If your attention starts to wander, return to the neutral nature of the lung meridian...

The lungs are dedicated organs, the weakest organ in our body… The lung is the first organ that a baby needs to activate after coming out of the mother's womb… the first thing after a child is born from a mother is to open the lobes of the lungs… crying is used to open the lobes of the lung.

The lung is the top source of five organs, is the first organ to feel the harm of the environment and the first organ to be affected by medications…

Know that after the meridian Qi returns to the lungs, the lungs will also distribute the twelve meridian Qi to the whole body… Understand that this kind of redistribution is strict, and it's not something any organ can have more than others… If the lung Qi is not descending, the quality of people's sleep will be poor.

Accept that the lungs are affected by grief, sadness and worry... People with severe skin problems also have grief, sadness and worry too… it doesn't matter how much topical medicine you put on skin, if the lung meridian has not been addressed, and the emotion has never been recognized and dealt with, the skin problem will never go away…

Always remember that you can avoid cold food and drinks, you can massage points along your lung meridian, but the absolute best way to protect your delicate lung meridian is to manage your emotions… and remember that an excellent tool to manage your emotions is meditation and mindfulness…

Fully understand that with practice, meditation itself can become the venue for manifesting and the discovery and development of you ... learning to observe yourself and your thoughts can be the first step toward moving away from powerless states of mind and a belief that external forces control you toward an empowered state of knowing yourself…

Set your intention to grow awareness of your power of meridian balance and harmony and understand that you can resist being carried along on a current not of your own making, resist blaming external forces for anything in your life, instead shaping your experience by setting your intention to achieve what you want and by extension affect your outer world experience…

Prepare for making the unconscious conscious through meditation, which will result in balanced meridians, enhanced focus, increased emotional intelligence, greater mental strength, improved physical health, healthy relationships and ultimately to self-realization…

Give yourself permission to embrace a new awareness of your power to create reality through the balancing of your meridians, through meditation and how this awareness will prepare you to live unconditionally...

Bring your awareness to the smile on your face as you realize that the meaning of life just may be to become who you came here to be and that becoming permeates your body, mind and soul...

Now that you are coming through all of this, notice the happiness you feel inside knowing how powerful meridian balance is and how connected to humanity you are...notice how this connection fills you with an elevated vibration... and how an elevated vibration can expand the visible spectrums of your senses...

Now just breathe and be with yourself and let the waves of your breathing be with you...

CHAPTER TWO

Large Intestine Meridian

Characteristics

The large intestine is the organ of transportation, it can transmit the dregs of food, make it change into feces and rid it from the body.

Known as the "Master of Transportation," it is the final organ before solid waste is eliminated.

From five am to seven am, meridian Qi mainly flows through the Large intestine meridian. If people wake up at that time, they should not consume caffeine, the body needs water; you should go for a brisk walk; if you wake up with an abdomen cramp and need to have a bowel movement then that means you have a healthy large intestine.

If not, then you can assist your large intestine meridian by drinking water. Drinking water prepares the body for the next meridian, which is the stomach meridian with Qi flow from seven am to nine am. This is the best time to have breakfast and this is the best way to take care of your digestion. This is the way of the meridian cycle, which is continuous as the Qi flows through the body.

The large intestine is in charge of making solid waste from liquid. It is the final organ before solid waste is eliminated.

The large intestine works closer with its paired organ than most. The lungs move the large intestine by breathing. The large intestine balances the body's fluids and works with the lungs in perspiration.

Large Intestine

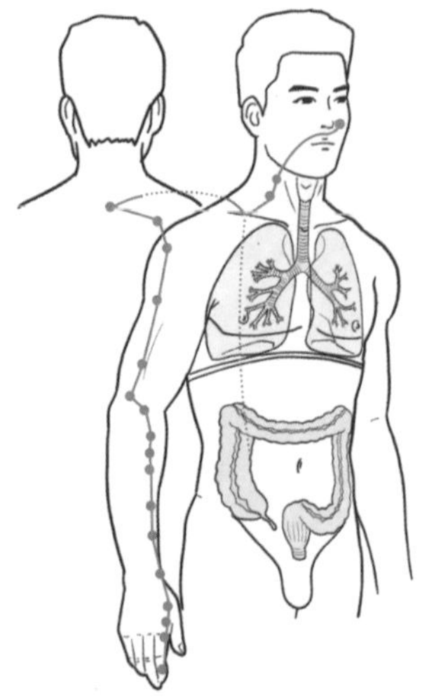

Primary Pathway

The Large Intestine Meridian starts from the tip of the index finger and runs between the thumb and the index finger.

It then proceeds along the lateral side of the forearm and the anterior side of the upper arm, until it reaches the highest point of the shoulder. From there, it has two branches.

One goes internally towards the lungs, diaphragm and large intestine.

The other travels externally upwards where it passes the neck and cheek, and enters the lower teeth and gums.

It then curves around the upper lip and crosses to the opposite side of the nose.

Both the lung meridian and the large intestine meridian take the index finger Shang Yang LI 1 point, where they are connected. The last point is Yingxiang LI 14, which is connected to the stomach meridian.

There are 20 points on one side of this meridian, 14 points on the radial side of the back of the arm, and 6 points on the shoulder, neck and face. Total 40 points on both side of the body .

Main Indications

An imbalance in the large intestine meridian can cause constipation, diarrhea, and abdominal pain. Depression and excessive worry can also be caused by an imbalance of this meridian.

Acupuncture points in this meridian are indicated for diseases affecting the head, face, pharynx (throat), febrile conditions and other symptoms along the meridian pathway.

Symptoms

Disharmony of the large intestine meridian can lead to symptoms of abdominal pain, intestinal cramping, diarrhea and constipation.

Toothache: Since this meridian passes through the oral cavity and the nose, symptoms like lower gum toothache, a runny nose, nosebleeds, and pain or heat along the meridian pathway can also indicate a disorder in this meridian.

Swollen neck and swollen cheeks are also problems with the large intestine meridian. At this time, scraping the large intestine meridian on the neck can be very effective.

Thyroid problem: The initial onset of thyroid disease also has the problem of neck swelling, which is generally related to the failure to completely cure the inflammation in the past. In addition, after profuse sweating, the human body is insufficiently healthy. Therefore, before thyroid disease, some people have cold or allergy problems all year round. As the neck muscles become more and more tense, it will lead to swelling of the thyroid gland. For this problem, you can use a Gua Sha board to scrape from the chin to the shoulders, and to the elbow along the large intestine line. It might be very painful, but keep doing it, it will help thyroid problems.

Constipation: the human body is actually a cavity. It has to facilitate entering and exiting. If you execute eating and defecating smoothly you will have no problems. Observing poop every day is also an important thing. If your child has a fever, don't keep staring at their head. As long as their bowel movements are smooth, it means that the inner movement is still normal, and the fever will gradually go away.

The large intestine meridian is also a meridian with very sufficient yang Qi, and constipation is caused by dryness and fire in Yangming. Diarrhea means dryness and decay of fire, so it hurts the body more than constipation.

In Chinese medicine, the stomach and the large intestine are like the two ends of a cavity. One tube goes in and the other tube goes out. Without going proper in and out, life will stagnate.

TCM Large intestine organ

As noted, the large intestine is the organ of transportation, it transmits the dregs of food and changes it into feces, ridding it from the body.

The intestine refers to the digestive tract from the pylorus of the stomach to the anus. The intestine is the longest section of the digestive tract and the most important part of the whole digestive function. The intestines of mammals include the small intestine, large intestine, and rectum. A large amount of digestion and the absorption of almost all foods are carried out in the small intestine. The large intestine mainly concentrates food residues to form feces, which are then excreted through the rectum and then through the anus.

The large intestine, carrying, changing, and transporting the human body's "trash" must be smooth; the small intestine, carrying, changing, and transporting the essence of the human body, must also be smooth. If you only regard them as "transmission," you may not be able to fully and profoundly understand them.

Remember, the lungs are the prime ministers of the whole body. The large intestine and lungs are in the same family. The two are congenital husband and wife, and the lungs dominate their worries so that the large intestine can be happy. When things are out of control or life is chaotic, the large intestine and its associated systems will have a problem; when you are overly stressed or encounter fear, the large and small intestines and their associated systems will have bigger problems.

In short, the large and small intestines must not only carry, transport and facilitate transformation in the human body, they must also carry the accumulation of our emotions.

Regarding emotions, Western medicine has terms for body chemistry: "dopamine" which produces pleasure, "norepinephrine" which brings passion, "endorphins" which are responsible for pleasure and pain relief, and "oxytocin" which helps us overcome difficulties and many more.

For example, if you have a very good time and are happy for the whole day, by the end of day you still feel very happy, this feeling is caused by dopamine. You have been busy for a day, very tired, and getting off work makes you feel happy. This feeling is caused by endorphins.

Western medicine believes that endorphins can fight pain, invigorate the spirit, and relieve depression; they can also allow us to resist grief, flourish creativity, improve work efficiency, be full of love and create a sense of light, positive, and willingness to communicate and collude with people around us.

Where do endorphins come from? Westerners believe that endorphins originate from the brain, and there are several ways to release endorphins:

1) Exercise. When the amount of exercise exceeds a certain period, the body will secrete endorphins. Therefore, if we can maintain half an hour of exercise every day, we can increase our happiness;

2) Certain foods, such as spicy flavor, can create painful sensations on the tongue. In order to balance this pain, the human body secretes endorphins to eliminate the pain on the tongue while creating a feeling similar to happiness in the human body. In addition, dark chocolate and ginseng can produce this pleasure;

3) Singing loud songs also contributes to the production of endorphins;

4) Good social activities or gardening work;

5) Love and sex, etc. These can make people produce "pleasure hormones" or "youth hormones" and keep people young and happy.

But from the theory of Tibetan chakras and Taoist practice, we can find that the deepest emotions actually originate from the bottom of the person's root chakra rather than the head.

For example, the root chakra is the intersection of life and death, fear, insecurity, pain, confusion. And the reproductive chakra is related to desire and possessiveness, creative desire, passion, willfulness, guilt, and abstinence.

Traditional Chinese medicine believes that Dantian is the birthplace of the fundamental desire of life. From this, we can infer that enkephalins may be derived from endorphins, that is, the happiness above comes from below. Good food, singing entertainment, sex, etc. can activate the central veins of the human body from bottom to top, thereby producing a feeling of happiness. At the very least, natural encephalins are found in the brain, spinal cord, and intestines.

This is probably also the true connotation of the large intestine as "the official of the transportation" in the Internal Classic. Transportation is not only the material level, it also refers to the spiritual level. In other words, whether we are happy or not is closely related to endorphin, and psychological disorders such as worry, depression, interpersonal tension, sleep disorders, etc. are all related to gastrointestinal dysfunction.

Modern Western science has also discovered that the intestines and stomach can be called the second brain of a person. Scientists have shown that the intestines and stomach contain not only a large number of nerve cells, but also a large number of microbes composed of bacteria. They will have an important impact on the human body's nervous system, especially the emotional regulation of joy, anger and sorrow, which in turn affects decision-making ability.

Acupoints

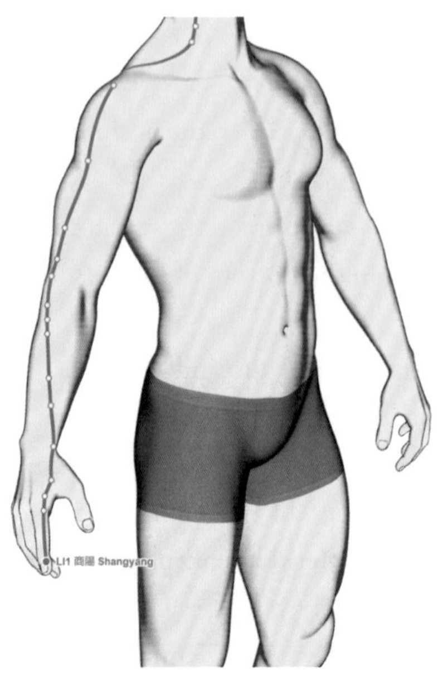

LI - 1 SHANG YANG (METAL'S NOTE YANG)

Name: Metal's Note Yang, Shang is the sound of metal. Open's the orifices, ears, nose and throat.

Location: on the posterior to the corner of the index fingernail.

Indication: Mainly treat sore throat and toothache, fever, coma, numbness at the index finger, and neck swelling.

Techniques and notes: Children with tonsil inflammation, or fever, can use a lancet to bleed it with LI - 1.

Constipated, you can use the Gua Sha board to scrape the index finger and the outside of the pinky finger separately, from the root of the finger to the tip of the finger, and Acupressure on the Shangyang, which can promote intestinal movement.

Shang Yang is also an important acupuncture point for male sexual function health care. It is commonly used to massage this acupoint with the thumb and fingertips, which has the obvious effect of strengthening yang, and can delay sexual aging.

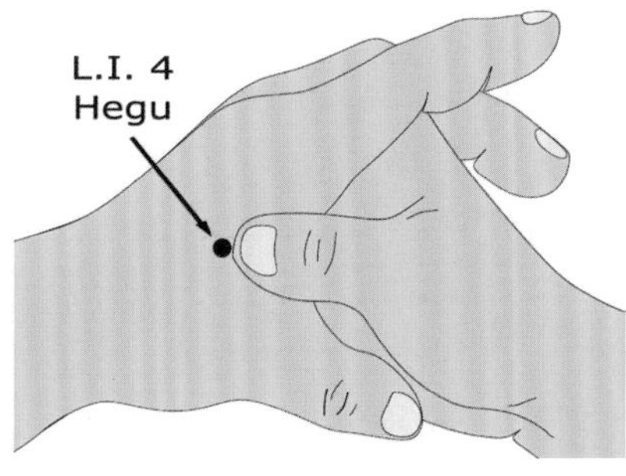

LI - 4 HE GU (UNION VALLEY)

Name: Union Valley, Valley like depression between the first and second metacarpal bones. Gu points also refers to transformation and relates to digestion.

Location: on the dorsum of the hand, between the 1st and 2nd metacarpal bones, at the approximate midpoint on the radial side of the 2nd metacarpal bone.

Indication: It is a special effect point for treating diseases of the head and face. This acupoint is a great point, and it has a strong force for activating the meridians, relaxing muscles and joints. It can treat pain, numbness, coldness, fever, paralysis, etc. in the parts of the large intestine meridian along the meridian.

Techniques and notes:

Gua Sha: Eczema, when eczema starts, you can scrape Gua Sha around He Gu for 5 minutes. Generally, the eczema will be relieved as soon as the bruised color comes out, and if you scrape two more times, the less severe eczema will basically heal. At the same time, add Gua Sha (scraping) Qu chi L.I 11 acupoint, which can relieve itching faster.

Acupressure: He Gu is the most stimulating point of the whole body reaction, which can lower blood pressure and calm nerves. Press this point with the thumb for one to three minutes each time. Strong stimulation of He Gu point can cure the inability to flex and extend the thumb and index finger. Hegu acupoint also can improve digestion function, and are good for headache, deafness, blurred vision, insomnia, neurasthenia etc.

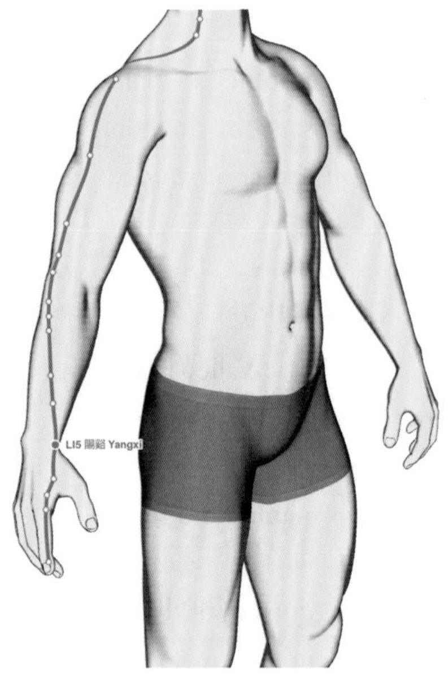

LI 5: YANG XI (YANG RAVINE)

Name: Yang Ravine, refers to depression between the two tendons, Xi refers back to the Kidneys (K - 3 Tai Xi), summon Yang Qi of Kidney to help the body to move inertia and wind cold.
Location: On the upper edge of the wrist, with the thumb extended, in the depression between the tendons of extensor pollicus longus and brevis.
Indication: Quit smoking
Technique and notes: pressure Yangxi Point for 3 minutes can reduce the desire to smoke

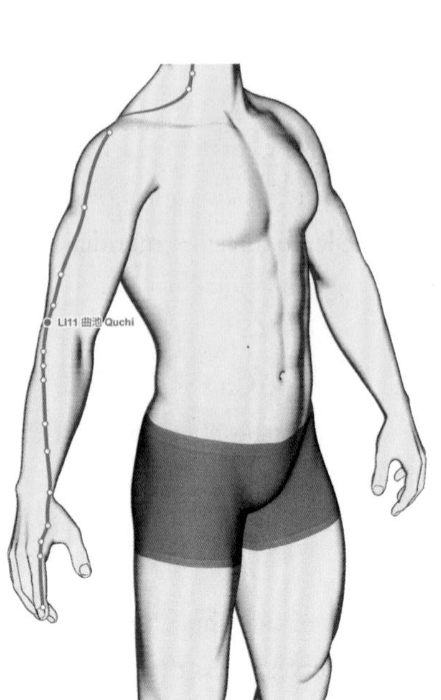

LI 11: QU CHI (POOL AT THE BEND)

Name: Pool at the Bend, accumulation of Qi nourishment at elbow.
Location: When the arm is flexed at elbow, the point is found at the lateral end of the transverse crease, midway between Lg-5 & the lateral epicondyle of the humorous.
Indication: is clinically mainly used for the treatment of arm pain, upper limb discomfort, fever, high blood pressure, anger; abdominal pain, vomiting and diarrhea, sore throat, toothache, red eyes, swelling and pain, addiction, eczema, scrofula, etc.
Technique and notes: Acupressure.
Gua Sha: When you have fever, colds, cough, or asthma, you can use a

Gua Sha board to scrape. If a bruised color is discharged, it can quickly relieve and reduce the fever.

Moxibustion can be used for 10 minutes.

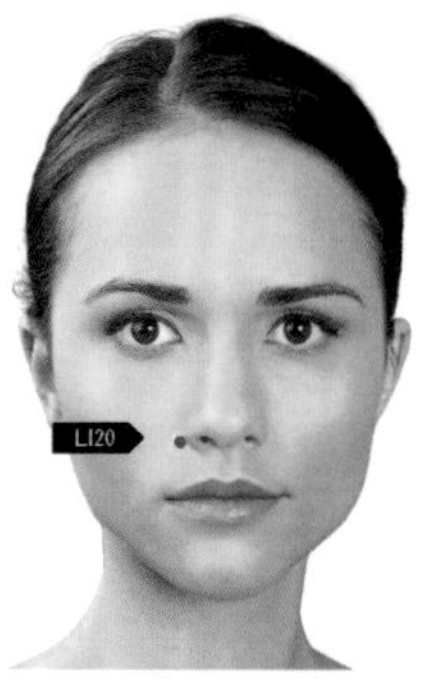

LI 20: YING XIANG (WELCOME FRAGRANCE)

Name: Welcome Fragrance, cannot smell because of nasal congestion.
Location: in the nasolabial groove, at the level of the midpoint of the lateral part of the nasal wing.
Indication: It is the main point for the treatment of various nose diseases; this point is the intersection point of the Large Intestine and Stomach Meridian. It can regulate the Qi of the two meridians and relieve the wind and heat of the two meridians. It is an important point for the treatment of various facial diseases: runny nose, nasal congestion, or allergic rhinitis caused by cold, massaging Ying Xiang can relieve symptoms immediately.
Technique and Notes: Acupressure.
How to look at health from the hand:
1) Look at the color, whether it is pink or not.
2) See if it is warm. Warm hands and feet are an important indicator of good health.
3) Check whether the pads of the finger are full and elastic. Wrinkled and inelastic fingers pads mean spleen deficiency.
4) Feel the pulsation of the fingertips whether it is active or not, which depends on the strength of the heart's blood vessels.

Miscellaneous bits:

Element: Metal
Direction: West
Season: Autumn

Climate: Dry
Sense Organ: Nose
Sense: Smell
Tissue: Skin and Hair
Positive Emotion: Courage
Negative Emotion: Grief
Flavor: Pungent (Umami)
Color: Off-White
Sound: Crying
Smell: Rotten
Time: 5 a.m. – 7 a.m.
Opposite: Kidney
Yin/Yang: Yang
Flow Direction: Down
Origin/Ending: Hand to Face
Number of Acupoints: 20 on one side of the body, 40 on both side.

Large Intestine Meditation

Resting comfortably now.

Feeling safe, calm, and at ease.

I want you, to give yourself permission, to take this time, just for you.

I want you to relax, and just for a little while at least, I want you to let go.

Let go of all the thoughts of responsibility that would normally preoccupy your mind.

Remember how good it is just to breathe properly and how calm it makes you feel.

Short pause.

You may feel a pleasant tingling in the nostrils as you breathe in through the nose and a loosening of tension as you breathe out from the mouth.

As you breathe in you begin to feel more and more comfortable, more and more relaxed and at ease.

You feel even more relaxed as you breathe out and you can allow the stomach rest as it wants to.

And you are breathing comfortably in and relaxing more as you breathe out.

Concentrate on your regular breathing.

The more you do this the more relaxed you become.

When you tense parts of the body and then relax them, you realize how comfortable it is to just tense and relax.

And the more comfortable you are, the more relaxed you feel.

Let us begin with the feet.

Tense the muscles in the toes and feet,

Now relax them.

Tense the shins.

Relax them.

Good.

Now tense the calf muscle and relax.

Tense the knees and relax.

Tense the thighs and relax and breathe comfortably in and relaxingly out.

Tense the muscles at the base of the spine.

Relax. Tense the tummy, and relax even further.

Tense the muscles of your chest.

Then just let go.

Tense the shoulders and then allow that tension to slump away…

Tense the neck, the chin, cheeks and facial muscles, tense all the little muscles around the eye,

That's good ...

Then go deeper within.

Go still deeper; go deep within your body, underneath the skin, inside those internal organs, inside your blood.

Travel along the Large Intestine Meridian which starts from the tip of the index finger and runs between the thumb and the index finger… follow along as it then proceeds along the lateral side of the forearm and the anterior side of the upper arm… until it reaches the highest point of the shoulder.

From there, it has two branches. One goes internally towards the lungs, diaphragm and large intestine ... The other travels externally upwards where it passes the neck and cheek, and enters the lower teeth and gums. It then curves around the upper lip and crosses to the opposite side of the nose.

Go deeper now within cells and still deeper within the atoms that form them.

And you can imagine this universe is deep within you.

Short pause.

As you go deeper into this universe, its infinite depth, deeper within yourself, you are pleased to feel more at home, more relaxed.

This is where you want to be.

Short pause.

Find yourself entering your own deep inner place; the place where you really want to be.

Each exhale deepens your relaxation tenfold.

You are feeling deeper and deeper relaxed.

And you realize that you are even more relaxed; you are ten times more again.

You are going ten times deeper and more relaxed than ever before.

You find yourself in this safe calm, inner place, familiar places that make you feel good and well as part of this experience.

You know that there will be everything you need, just to be.

You realize you are easily in control, of this inner place - of yourself - and your body.

You can regulate your breathing, without too much effort and breathing will naturally become slow and easy.

You know how to do this as you have done it before. In comfortable - out relax.

You can control the outer body to reflect a calm presence.

Your heart rate can be slowed if needed.

No longer is there any need to worry about being alone with stress or anxiety as this home is always within.

You are in control in this secure inner place deep, deep within yourself, where outside worries don't matter.

The confidence and calm of this place will always be with you, because you now have the knowledge that you can come to this inner place at any time, from any place as it is always within you.

To revisit this inner place, simply clench the right hand into a fist and the stretch out the fingers, resting them as you say to yourself the words, inner place. Do all this three distinct times.

The calm control will then immediately take effect as you feel yourself releasing tension and going back to that inner place.

To return to your normal state you will simply say "back 1, 2, 3" or just return to your normal state after 15 or twenty minutes.

Now that you have a better understanding of yourself and found new ways of dealing with the world in general, you are going to feel much more at peace and so much calmer than before… You can apply this technique to the balance of your chakras, to the harmony of your meridians…

On a subtle level you understand… all the parts of your body are made of molecules, atoms and sub-atomic particles, and these are in constant motion… Try to really get a feeling for the change that is taking place each moment in your body…. This will help you begin to understand Qi…

Feel how your awareness of your meridians empowers you to alter your body's balance; how your meridian awareness can provide the opportunity to not only shift from wherever you are to balance and harmony, but also to project love and kindness to others…

Embrace the fact that over the course of 2,500 years, Traditional Chinese Medicine has become a tried and tested system of rational medicine known for its great diversity of healing and wellness practices ... know that the main goal of TCM is to create harmony between our mind, body, and the environment around us...

Know that oftentimes, physical symptoms can be made worse by, or even result from, an imbalance of energy in your body rather than an issue in the particular spot where you are experiencing discomfort ... understand that health is all about balance, and when it is thrown off, you become more susceptible to disease ... Energy is the director of your body's harmony; its movement is crucial to your health...

Understand too that one very important way to create harmony is by making sure your Qi is balanced ... Qi means life energy and it stands for the energy in all things...

From the theory of Tibetan chakras and Taoist practice, we can find that the deepest emotions actually originate from the bottom of the person's root chakra rather than from the head ... the root chakra is the intersection of life and death, fear, insecurity, pain, confusion ... the reproductive chakra is related to desire-possessiveness and possessiveness, creative desire, passion, willfulness, guilt, and abstinence ... the Dantian is the birthplace of the fundamental desire of life.... the happiness above comes from below.

Good food, singing entertainment, sex, and so much more activates the central veins of the human body from bottom to top, thereby producing a feeling of happiness ... learn to produce happiness from your inner journeys...

Journey along the large intestine as the official of transportation... Transportation not only at the material level, but also the spiritual level ... happiness or unhappiness is closely related to endorphins, and psychological disorders such as worry, depression, interpersonal tension, sleep disorders, etc. are all related to gastrointestinal dysfunction ... journey inward along the official of transportation to make your large intestine happy and in so doing make yourself happy...

Pause...

When you return in a few moments to the here and now after this session bring back with you new insights - new learning's, new possibilities and new avenues for you to explore.

Pause…

Connect presently in this meditation on an energetic level now… form an energetic circle of connection,… send love outward now… send that loving sensation out to larger and larger circles of others forming a unified connection with your fellow humans and the universe...

Now that you have come through this meditation, notice how you feel in your body… how happy you feel… Take a moment to take three slow, deep breaths and feel how wonderful it is to live a life filled with happiness…

Now just breathe and be present with yourself for a moment, and then come back when you are ready…

CHAPTER THREE

Stomach Meridian

Characteristics

The stomach meridian is the longest meridian on the front side of the human body.

The stomach is the Sea of Nourishment. This sea contains hundreds of rivers and transforms everything.

Also known as the Minister of the Mill, it is the start of digestion. The umbilical cord influences the referral to the stomach meridian as the Root of Postnatal Life.

From seven am to nine am, meridian Qi mainly flows through the stomach meridian, this is the best time to have breakfast. Breakfast needs to include good protein and other foods that provide for good energy. People who have stomach problems need to have a good breakfast during this time. This is the way of the meridian cycle, which is continuous as the Qi flows through the body.

The stomach is in charge of elemental balance and is referred to, as noted above, the Sea of Nourishment; this sea contains hundreds of rivers and transforms everything, good and bad. All can be melted away.

The stomach is tasked with extracting the energy from food and beverages. Working with the spleen, the stomach transports the energy throughout the meridian system. The stomach also uses the different types of food eaten to balance the five elemental energies.

If a person is tall, has plump cheeks, a thick neck, and a broad chest, it indicates that his stomach energy is strong. A long nose indicates that the condition of the large intestine is good. The lips are thick and the philtrum is deep, indicating a good small intestine.

As the minister of the mill, the stomach is the origin of the five flavors. In TCM, flavors share the names of the different tastes we perceive on our palate (bitter, sour, salty, pungent, and sweet). In the Chinese methodology, each flavor also signals a food's therapeutic effect upon the body's systems. The botanical world gives us a full palette of flavors for supporting health.

The five flavors on the surface are distinguished by the tongue, and the tongue is the sense organ related to the heart. The inner five flavors are distinguished by the stomach. Therefore, loss of taste is both a heart condition as well as a stomach condition.

With the skillful application of the five flavors to balance the phases and the corresponding organs and channels, the body can return to harmony and health.

One of the primary problems for people within the COVID experience was the loss of smell and taste. Where is the problem? The lung Qi flows through the nose. If the lungs are in harmony, the nose can recognize the smell; if the lungs are not in harmony, the nose cannot distinguish the five smells, and the smell will not be smelled, so the sense of smell is related to the lungs.

If the heart is not in harmony, the tongue cannot distinguish the five flavors because the tongue is the sense organ related to the heart. In fact, the sense of taste is closely related to the sense of smell. For example, when you have a cold, if you lose your sense of smell, you will not taste anything when you eat. It can be seen that smell and taste are inseparable. So, when the heart, spleen and stomach have problems, the sense of taste will have problems.

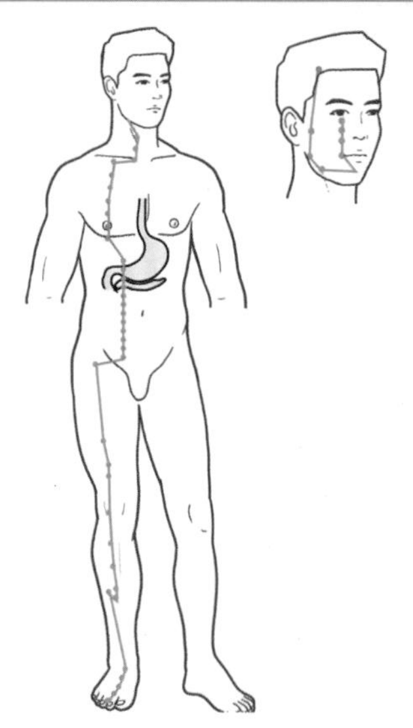

Primary Pathway

There are 45 points on one side of the foot Yang Ming of the Stomach Meridian and 90 points on the left and right sides.

Among them, there are eight acupuncture points on the face and head, almost covering the face.

The stomach meridian belongs to Yang Ming, which is a meridian of more Qi and blood. Compared with other meridians, the stomach meridian transports more blood and Qi to the head.

Since it's a long meridian, I will explain one section at time so that everyone can have better understanding.

The Stomach Meridian starts from the end of the Large Intestine Meridian at the side of the nose, which is the end point of the large intestine meridian. This is evidence of the connection between the stomach and the large intestine. You can see that people have an image when they are old, that is, there are wrinkles on the upper lip which is a sign of the decline of the large intestine. It means that there is a problem with the communication between the stomach and the large intestine.

The meridian passes through the inner corner of the eye to emerge from the lower part of the eye. Going downwards, it enters the upper gum and curves around the lips and lower jaw.

The stomach meridian connects with the bladder meridian at the beginning of eyebrow Jing Ming and connects with the small intestine meridian at the end of the eyebrow. Therefore, when you look at the eyebrows, it is entirely a manifestation of Yang Qi, the beginning of brows is the bladder meridian; the middle of the eyebrows is the stomach meridian; the end of the eyebrows is the small intestine meridian. So the taller and thicker the eyebrows, the more Yang Qi, the more the person loves to take care of things. The woman's eyebrows that are light but curvy mean they have grateful and leisurely personalities.

The whole outside of the nose is all part of the stomach meridian, so anything that grows on the nose is a matter of the stomach meridian. Many people have blackheads on their noses, or they have very large pores on both sides of the nose, which is a cold stomach. The pimples are mostly found on the stomach meridians on the face, such as around the forehead, cheeks and nose, so they also belong to stomach meridian conditions.

Pimples on foreheads, cheeks and noses all point to cold stomach.

The meridian flows into the upper teeth. Problems with the upper teeth are all problems with the stomach meridian. The lower gum problem is with the large intestine.

The stomach meridian protrudes from the upper teeth, is held on both sides of the mouth, surrounds the lips, and intersects left and right at the Cheng Jiang point of the chin and lip groove. The large intestine meridian also circles around the mouth and the lips, so the bumps and pimples that surround the lips are a gastrointestinal problem, as well as a weakened immune system.

The more raised the chin, the greater the blessing of a person.

It then turns upwards, passing in front of the ear, until it reaches the corner of the forehead where it splits into an internal and external branch. In short, the corner of the forehead is all about the stomach meridian. As long as your eyebrows and forehead hurt, it is a stomach problem.

The external branch crosses the neck, chest, abdomen and groin where it goes further downward along the front of the thigh and the lower leg, until it reaches the top of the foot.

The internal branch emerges from the lower jaw, running downwards until it reaches its pertaining organ, the stomach.

The meridian crosses the neck and so it affects the throat area. Dry throat can be caused from the stomach fire or heat.

At the chest, the meridian passes the nipples and breast area. Itchy nipples belong to the cold stomach. Let's talk about breasts. What are breasts? It is a storage warehouse for women's blood. Breast milk is the production of stomach blood. The size of the breast is determined by the Chong Mai (Sea of Blood), which is one of the extraordinary meridians. The amount of blood and milk depends on how much the stomach can transform, not the size of the breast. Some people have small breasts, but the milk is very strong, indicating that she has a strong ability to transmit blood from food.

Then go down, into the knee patella. So the problem of the knee is the problem of the stomach meridian, such as patellar softening, which is a stomach meridian disease.

There is a simple way to protect your knees: spread your five fingers, cover the knee joints with your palms, and gently rub and massage your knee joints. Do this five to ten minutes per day.

Additionally, the kneeling method is a good method to exercise the stomach meridian. Kneel down and crawl on a carpeted floor. After the knee is squeezed, it will promote more blood and Qi around knee joints. It's a very direct way to bring knee blood circulation back. In the beginning, take your time, start slowly, a few minutes at a time, and slowly walk forward on your knees. Basically, your knee pain will decrease as you can kneel longer.

Finally, it terminates at the lateral side of the tip of the second toe. Another branch emerges from the top of the foot and ends at the big toe to connect with the Spleen Meridian.

The stomach meridian goes through the chest and breasts, all the way to the Qi Jie point (groin area) at the base of the thigh. As long as there is a problem along the path of the stomach meridian, it will be treated from the stomach. Any swelling and pain along the path of the meridian is a gastric disease, including swelling of the instep and the inability to flex and extend the middle toe.

Main Indication

Acupuncture points in this meridian are indicated for certain gastro enteric diseases, toothaches and mental illnesses. Conditions that affect areas through which the meridian passes such as the head, face, eyes, nose and mouth can also benefit from stimulation of the acupuncture points along this meridian.

Symptoms

An imbalance with the stomach meridian will cause energetic deficiencies across the Meridian System. It can also cause mania, confusion, or anxiety, stomach ache, rapid digestion, hunger, nausea and vomiting, or thirst.

Other symptoms that relate to disorders along the meridian pathway include abdominal distension, ascites (a fluid buildup in the abdomen), sore throat, nosebleeds, or pain in the chest or knee.

Following are some common symptoms related to the stomach that people might not be aware that are related to the stomach:

Yawning all the time. This is a lack of stomach Qi. It is good to take the initiative to yawn and stretch when you wake up in the morning. However, within 5-10 days before the onset of ischemic stroke, the patient will also yawn frequently. It is possible that cerebral arteriosclerosis is gradually getting worse, the lumen is getting narrower, and the performance of cerebral ischemia and hypoxia is aggravated, which is the sign of imminent stroke. This is an important alarm signal. If you are choking while eating, or even swallow saliva, you have to check your brain or lungs.

Hiccups.

The corners of the foreheads are dark. If it's kidney problems then the whole forehead is completely dark.

Tibia skin numbness and muscle tingling which is a sign of the malfunction of the stomach.

Anemia. Commonly, people take iron supplementation for this condition. In fact, if you want to completely solve the problem of being anemic, you must start with the spleen and stomach. When the spleen and stomach are sufficient, people can have the ability to produce blood.

Many people have a crooked mouth when they smile. Spleen and stomach problems are to blame because of the stomach meridian circle around the mouth.

Bloating, swelling and pain in the legs and knees. Stomach meridian syndrome will manifest in the swelling of the abdomen and legs, as well as swelling and pain of the knees. So the best way to exercise the stomach meridian is the “kneeling method” mentioned earlier.

Eat large portions and get hungry again fast. At the same time, the urine becomes yellow, which is unfavorable for absorption, causing the absorption of the subtle flow away diminishing stomach heat and fire.

Bloating and feeling full after eating when the stomach is cold. Cold in the stomach means that the stomach Qi does not condense. I see too many patients with this problem now, the stomach is bloated after eating, all sorts of discomforts, in other words, the stomach is cold and cannot digest the food. People who use digestive enzymes or probiotics still have problems; warming stomach herbs are still needed. The key is warm the stomach!

Depression and Anxiety. The stomach meridian off balance can cause mental problems. Many manifestations of depression are connected to lack of stomach Qi and Yang energy.

Is it any wonder that there is an epidemic of depression and anxiety in our country today given that what we eat is referred to as the Standard American Diet (SAD)? We eat the wrong things at the wrong times and wonder why we don’t feel right. The answer from allopathic medicine is pills, which besides having terrible side effects, even when they work properly all that they are doing is masking the symptoms. Chemical therapy does NOT get to the root of the problem, which is stomach meridian Qi and Yang energy balance.

Many people don’t know that the stomach meridian being off balance can cause mental problems. Don’t underestimate the impact of stomach problems and a cold stomach. All mania and depression can be cured from the stomach.

Symptoms of depression and anxiety include being afraid of seeing people, sensitive to light and, or loud noise, like to be alone, pessimistic, lacking self-confidence. These symptoms can be attributed to lacking stomachs Qi and Yang.

Depression and anxiety are rampant in our society today. A friend is a high school teacher in Santa Cruz. He told me that every one of his students is on antidepressants.

As with any medication, it hurts the stomach the most. The reason so many children are on medication right now is that many parents are also very anxious and depressed, too. The most important thing for a child is vitality, which is a powerful self-healing state. The reason for this reference resource is to teach and educate on the power and availability of self-healing.

In terms of treatment, we must first understand that this syndrome is generally in the Yin meridian.

The overall treatment principle is: break the stomach cold, clear the meridians, and replenish the essence and blood.

To break the stomach cold, you can use traditional Chinese medicine, moxibustion Zhongwan or Guan Yuan. The meridian energy becomes opened, balanced and cleared and the essence and blood become naturally sufficient

How to nourish the stomach?

Avoid getting angry, manage emotions, love and happiness can nourish the stomach the most.

Avoid mixing too many different kinds of foods in each meal.

Take less medicines and chemical anti-inflammatories; these are most likely to cause cold conditions in the lungs, stomach, and kidneys because all the chemicals are cold in nature.

Do not drink cold drinks. Have warm soup frequently.

Be quiet when eating.

Eat slowly and chew 20 times at each bite.

The stomach is the second face of a person. For example, when others accuse you, you may have a gentle smile on your face, but the stomach has already convulsed and contracted. Therefore, the stomach holds not only food, but also love and anger.

Stomach disease is related to the following situations:

Eating too fast, or talking while eating. Chewing slowly is not only good for the stomach, but also beauty.

Anger and depression, especially the stress at family relationships are the worst thing for the stomach.

Cold drinks. Drink warm to room temp water. Especially in summer, the sun heats the body surface, so the inside of our body is cold, too many cold drinks will deplete stomach Yang. We need to pay attention, either no or few cold drinks in summer.

Overeating.

Over nutrition or malnutrition.

When desires are inconsistent with reality, it can cause acid reflux and stomach ulcer.

Nowadays, there are more people with discomfort in the stomach. Too many thoughts hurt digestion, spleen and stomach as do anger and depression. When the ideal is not in line with reality, the stomach acid is reversed. Maintaining a healthy stomach and spleen requires less thought and managing emotions and stress. Let happiness dissolve everything!

Your appetite affirms the relationship between food and desire.

Appetite is not only a problem of hunger and fullness. It sometimes stems from our deep desire or unconscious emptiness.

Eating can be very emotional.

Some people eat because of loneliness, some people eat because of emptiness. The fullness that comes from this emotional eating is still not satisfying, but instead leads to a deep sense of self-pity and possession of a certain material security.

And some people have no appetite, not just because of the lack of energy in the stomach and digestion, but because of disgust and nausea towards reality.

When eating is carried out for any other reason than nourishment, the stomach meridian is moved away from balance.

Acupoints

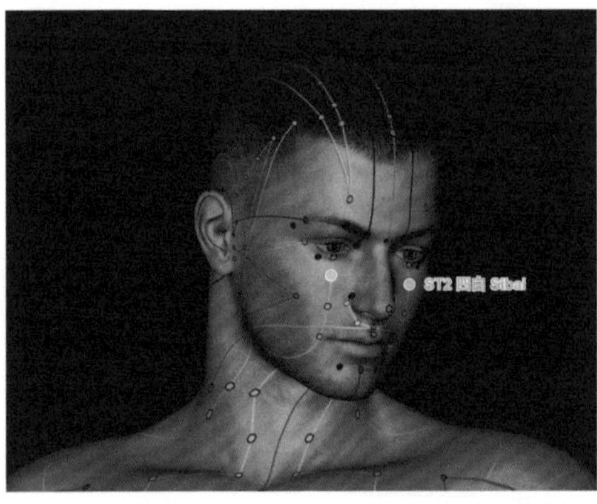

ST 2: SI BAI (FOUR WHITE)

Name: Four White, the four white areas, above, below and to the sides of the iris. Clearing the sight in all four directions.
Location: one cm (finger) below the pupil of the eye, in the depression at the infraorbital foramen.
Indication: Brightens the eyes, any eye issues, facial paralysis, acupuncture face lifts.
Techniques and notes: Acupressure or Gua Sha. The best easy way is to use Gua Sha board to scrape from Si Bai along the cheek bones to the front of the ear.

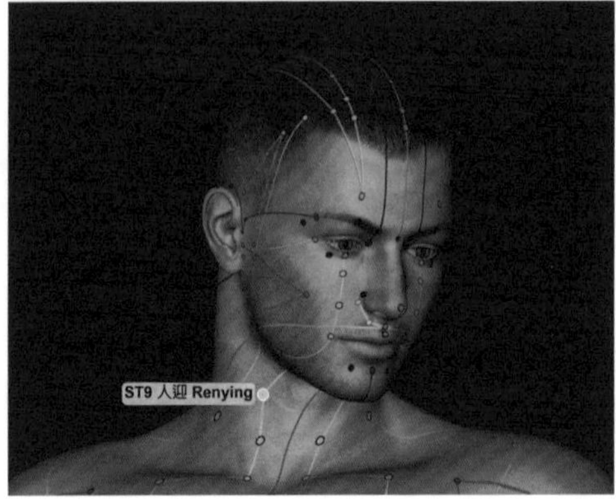

ST 9: REN YING (MAN'S WELCOME)

Name: Man's Welcome: To have the ability to receive and express. To open to our higher possibilities and let go of hurt. To be able to accept what earth/life has given you.
Location: On the anterior artery border m. sternocleidomastoids, 1.5 cun (one cun which is the width of your thumb) lateral to the laryngeal prominence.
Indication: mainly treats sore throat, asthma, scrofula, and high blood pressure.
Techniques and Notes: Moxibustion is not allowed here. But there must be frequent massage, and scraping.

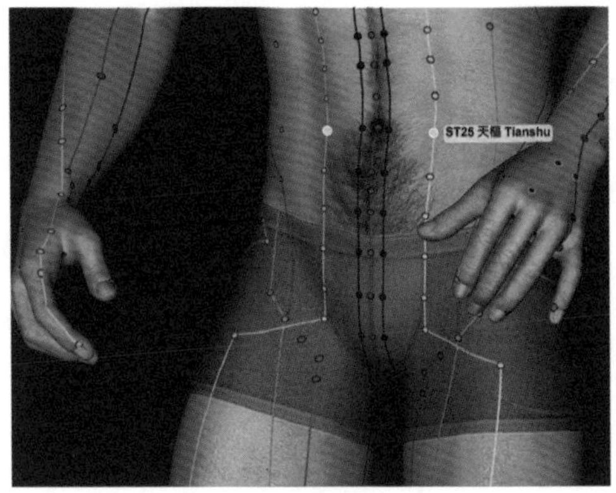

ST 25: TIAN SHU (CELESTIAL AXIS)

Name: Celestial Axis, the body's center that is the juncture of heavenly Qi and earthly Qi. The hub of heaven and earth, above the belly button is the sky, and below the belly button is the earth, so Tian Shu is particularly important. It is the reversal of heaven and earth, so he is in charge of the Qi machine, which can press, knead, acupuncture, and moxibustion, but pregnant women can't use moxibustion.

Location: In the middle of the abdomen, 2 cun lateral to the center of the umbilicus. The deep part is the small intestine.

Indication: diarrhea, abdominal cramping, acute and chronic gastritis, acute and chronic enteritis, appendicitis, intestinal paralysis, bacillary dysentery, indigestion, urinary calculi, irregular menstruation, appendicitis, endometritis, nephritis, edema, hypertension, low back pain, convulsions in children, intermittent fever, biliary ascariasis, etc.

Techniques and Notes: massage and moxibustion, stomach and intestinal diseases can all be helped by Tianshu. It is more effective to massage the belly and Tianshu at the same time. Even if you have a fever, especially when the upper body is hot and the lower body is cold, and no medicine is available, you can use moxibustion on each side of the Tian Shu.

In fact, the more we learn, the more we understand our body, we will have more tools to heal ourselves. After learning about the meridians, we understand what's going on with our body, we can massage the meridian. After we learned acupuncture points, we can acupressure the points. We will have less fear and worries.

QI JIE

Location: Just above the groin, 5 inches below the middle of the belly button, and 2 inches from the anterior midline.

Indications of bowel, abdominal pain, hernia, irregular menstruation, infertility, impotence, swelling of the vagina.

The Qi Jie point refers to the pulsation of the inguinal artery.

From here, go in and down to the uterus and ovaries, and then to the groin area at the base of the thighs. Breast and the uterus problems are related. As long as the stomach is cold, the breast must be cold and the uterus must be cold; as long as the uterus is cold, the stomach must be cold. Therefore, during menstruation, the stomach is cold and breasts are swollen and painful, and at the same time the thighs are sore. So don't drink cold beverages during menstruation.

The Qi Jie is related to both the Gallbladder Meridian- Chong Mai (extra meridian) and Stomach Meridian, and is a channel for transferring Qi. It is good for gynecology, men's prostate, etc. You pad this area, but you cannot use too much force. You can also use hot compresses here. Instead of spending a lot of money to go to a beauty salon for maintenance, it is better to pat yourself at home. When we were born, we had already let our hands droop naturally, and they were just placed on the Qi Jie acupoints, which means letting us massage and rub the Qi Jie to benefit the whole body, which means that we can help ourselves without asking for help.

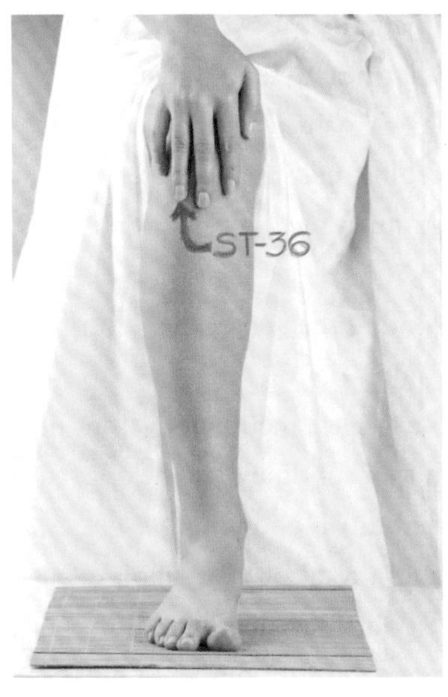

ST 36: ZU SAN LI (LEG THREE MILES)

Name: Leg Three Miles, this is a point that gives the stability and strength to walk an extra 3 miles. It is a large health point for the human body.
Location: On the anterior and outer side of the calf, 4 fingers below the calf's nose, and a horizontal one finger from the front edge of the tibia.
Indications: stomach pain, vomiting, choking, abdominal distension, diarrhea, dysentery, constipation, breast carbuncle, intestinal carbuncle, arthralgia of lower limbs, edema, madness, athlete's foot, as well as weight loss. Because the stomach controls blood diseases, it also treats dysmenorrhea. It also treats toothache above the stomach meridian.
Energetics: Tonifies the whole-body Qi and blood, immune system tonic, boosts vitality - to have the ability to do the things that you want to accomplish in life.
Techniques and notes: massage 3-5 mins each time.

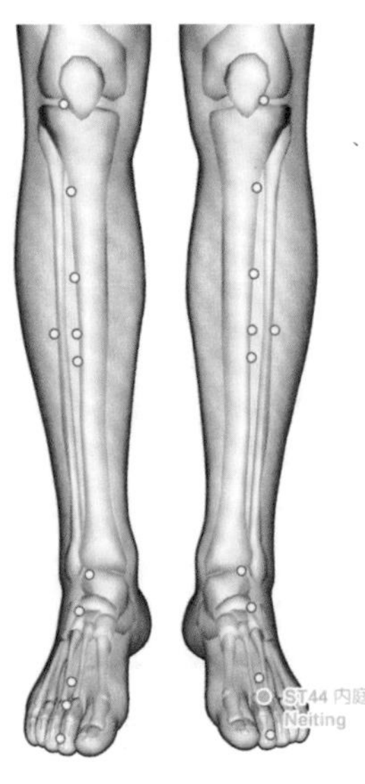

ST 44: NEITING (INNER COURTYARD)

Name: Inner Courtyard, anatomically, the courtyard represents the space between the toes, Nei is a person with a room. Heat effects the stomach channel causing shen disturbance and feeling of isolation.
Location: On the back of the foot, between the second toe and the third toe, in the depression distal and lateral to the second metatarsodigital joint.

Indications: it is used to treat upper tooth pain, throat swelling, crooked mouth, epistaxis, stomach acid, swelling, diarrhea, dysentery, constipation, fever, and back of the foot swelling and pain. Toothache, sore throat, stomach acid, bad breath, nose bleeding, constipation, etc. caused by stomach fire can be treated by stimulating and rubbing the inner court acupoints of both feet.

Techniques and notes: You can press the Neiting then enter the Lidui point outside the middle toe.

To sum up, the stomach meridian is the longest meridian in front of the human body. It has two main lines and four sub-lines, and belongs to the meridian with the most branches in the human body.

There are 45 acupoints on one side, and a total of 90 acupoints on the left and right sides. Among them, 15 points are distributed on the anterior and outer sides of the lower limbs, and 30 points are on the abdomen, chest, and head and face. Among them, they are extremely abundant on the head and face. They are important meridians for overall health and for beauty as well.

It can be said that the stomach meridian is the most important meridian in front of the human body, and the bladder meridian is the most important meridian behind the human body. These two meridians are of great significance to health preservation.

Miscellaneous bits:

Element: Earth
Direction: Center
Season: Late Summer
Climate: Damp
Sense Organ: Mouth
Sense: Taste
Tissue: Muscles
Positive Emotion: Compassion
Negative Emotion: Anxiety

Flavor: Sweet
Color: Yellow
Sound: Singing
Smell: Fragrant
Time: 7 a.m. – 9 a.m.
Opposite: Pericardium
Yin/Yang: Yang
Flow Direction: Down
Origin/Ending: Face to Foot
Number of Acupoints: 45 on each side for a total of 90

Stomach Meditation

Resting comfortably now.

Feeling safe, calm, and at ease.

I want you, to give yourself permission, to take this time, just for you.

I want you to relax, and just for a little while at least, I want you to let go.

I want you to just make yourself comfortable - as you listen to the sound of my voice. Softly close your eyes and slow your breathing…

And as you listen to me… you may be aware from time to time that your mind is beginning to wander… and if it does… that is fine… just let your own thoughts come and go as they will… because this is your time to relax - and true relaxation takes no effort at all.

During your everyday activities you are using a lot of muscle groups and energy and there is so much information filtering through your senses that it can make your body tense and strained… however taking the next few minutes to just be will allow you to unwind and let go of the cares of each day… so that when you return to the here and now you will feel totally refreshed, re-energized and alive - and able to deal more effectively with whatever you need to do ...

There is no time but now… there is no place but here… and right here… and right now… we are going to join in the sacred contemplation of what if… what if we could calm ourselves in any moment… what if we could settle our stomach chi and return to balanced yang energy on demand… let's go on a journey of discovery… a journey that can empower you to unwind from the cares of the day anytime you wish… for balance… for harmony…

Perhaps you can imagine your body as a raging ocean… your breathing is like the tempestuous waves on that ocean… rising up… falling down… ebbing and flowing… responding to weather patterns… the worries of the day are like a fierce gale force wind… as the great waves thrash against the sea wall… constantly raging… foaming and splashing against the jagged rocks… sending up fountains of frothy white sea spray...

The deep waters of your ocean contain countless of micro-organisms and a multitude of colorful, interesting sea-life… all of which have a part to play… just like the cells and organs and all systems of your body… supporting you as you support them ... like the stomach… also known as the sea of nourishment…

At times it can feel as though your body and mind have been ravaged by the storm - all the events of the day building up and up… and it is now time to rebalance yourself… tune out from the stresses and strains of modern-day life… and enjoy this quality time… allowing your body to rest and relax and tune into your inner place of peace and tranquility...

So, imagine now… that the storm is passing… the sky becomes brighter and bluer as the sun breaks through the clouds which disperse slowly and effortlessly away and over the far horizon...

You are your ocean… your body is resting, relaxing… breathing more slowly and evenly… all the muscles relaxing… easing away all the tensions of the day… feeling at peace with all the life in your ocean… which responds to the passing of the storm and the stillness that is all around you ... allowing your sea of nourishment to become the minister of the mill…

Let your body feel heavy and limp if you will - or allow it to float above the ocean to a place where you can gain a wider perspective of the life that is existing around you in such a calm way...

Your ocean is your sea of tranquility… a place where you can feel calm and relaxed and at peace with the universe ... Your relaxing thoughts and emotions bob about on top of the gently moving sea as the lapping waves edge slowly toward the safety of the shoreline...

Every cell, every consciousness, every nerve and fiber of your body are totally and completely relaxed ... You haven't a care in the world right now… nothing else matters but this wonderful feeling of relaxation.

And relaxation comes easy to you… because every day you make a point of spending some quality time… allowing your body and mind to relax… experience the storm of the day passing over… replaced by a calm, sunny day and your sea becomes tranquil and serene again… and when you come here… you can stay here until you are ready to return to the here and now… knowing that you will always arise feeling wonderfully refreshed and alert with your mind focused - and you are able to deal effectively with whatever you need to do ...

Now that you have a better understanding of how to use the imagery of the sea to reach an inner calm and found new ways of dealing with the world in general, you are going to feel much more at peace and so much calmer than before… You can apply this technique to the balance of your chakras, to the harmony of your meridians…

On a subtle level you understand… all the parts of your body are made of molecules, atoms and sub-atomic particles, and these are in constant motion… Try to really get a feeling for the change that is taking place each moment in your body…. This will help you begin to understand Qi…

Feel how your awareness of your meridians empowers you to alter your body's balance; how your meridian awareness can provide the opportunity to not only shift from wherever you are to balance and harmony, but also to project love and kindness to others…

Embrace the fact that over the course of 2,500 years, Traditional Chinese Medicine has become a tried and tested system of rational medicine known for its great diversity of healing and wellness practices ... know that the main goal of TCM is to create harmony between our mind, body, and the environment around us...

Know that oftentimes, physical symptoms can be made worse by, or even result from, an imbalance of energy in your body rather than an issue in the particular spot where you are experiencing discomfort ... understand that health is all about balance, and when it is thrown off, you become more susceptible to disease ... Energy is the director of your body's harmony; its movement is crucial to your health...

Understand too that one very important way to create harmony is by making sure your Qi is balanced ... Qi means life energy and it stands for the energy in all things...

Understand that the stomach is in charge of elemental balance ... as the sea of nourishment the stomach meridian maintains elemental balance when it is calm… leading to the sea are hundreds of rivers… and this sea metamorphoses everything, good and bad, all is melted away… but the balance and the melting are always better in a calm sea…

As the minister of the mill, the stomach meridian is the heart of digestion ... importantly, it is also home to the umbilical cord, which makes the stomach meridian the root of postnatal life ... the stomach meridian will rule your physical world for the rest of your life… nurturing it, keeping it calm… will impact your life in many ways…

The stomach meridian starts from the end of the large intestine meridian at the side of the nose, which is the end point of the large intestine meridian. This is evidence of the connection between the stomach and the large intestine. This meridian then flows all the way down to the foot…

Know that the stomach works with the spleen to transport energy throughout the Meridian System ... and the stomach uses the different types of food eaten to balance the five elemental energies ... visualize feeding the stomach nourishing foods at the right times for balance and harmony…

The minister of the mill is balanced by the five flavors ... The five flavors on the surface are distinguished by the tongue, and the tongue is the sense organ related to the heart; the inner five flavors are distinguished by the stomach ... perhaps you have heard that the way to a man's heart is through his stomach, but did you ever wonder why? We are connected in beautiful and harmonious ways… when we understand these ways of connections, these meridian maps… we can know a balance and harmony like never before…

Breathe in… and breathe out… breathe in… and breathe out… and with each breath that you take and with each word that is uttered perhaps you can feel your body relaxing… more and more.

I wonder if you can imagine yourself standing underneath a waterfall of relaxation… just feel that relaxing, comfortable feeling flowing all the way down your body.

All the way down from the top of your head to the tips of your toes… soothing, calming… relaxation… easing away any tensions.

Making you feel good… making you feel comfortable… making you feel so relaxed…

It is a wonderful feeling to be so relaxed… and quite perfect to be here right now - enjoying this calming, soothing experience...

When you return in a few moments to the here and now after this session bring back with you new insights - new learning's, new possibilities and new avenues for you to explore…

Pause…

Now that you have come through this meditation, notice how you feel in your body… how happy you feel… Take a moment to take three slow, deep breaths and feel how wonderful it is to live a life filled with happiness…

Now just breathe and be present with yourself for a moment, and then come back to the present when you are ready…

CHAPTER FOUR

Spleen Meridian

Characteristics

The Spleen meridian includes the pancreas and is involved in digestion. The spleen is referred to as the "Minister of the Granary." Nutrients from food and beverages are extracted by enzymes produced in the spleen and pancreas.

The spleen meridian regulates the quantity and the quality of blood in circulation and works with the lung meridian to generate True Human Energy. This meridian is affected by the tone of muscles and affects them in turn. The spleen meridian is responsible for logical and analytical thinking. It is also the first meridian in memory formation.

From nine am to eleven am, meridian Qi mainly flows through the Spleen meridian, this is the best time to work and be active.

Do your most taxing tasks of the day at this time.

The spleen meridian is referred to as the Minister of the Granary. Nutrients from food and beverages are extracted by enzymes produced in the spleen and pancreas. The meridian regulates the quantity and the quality of blood in circulation.

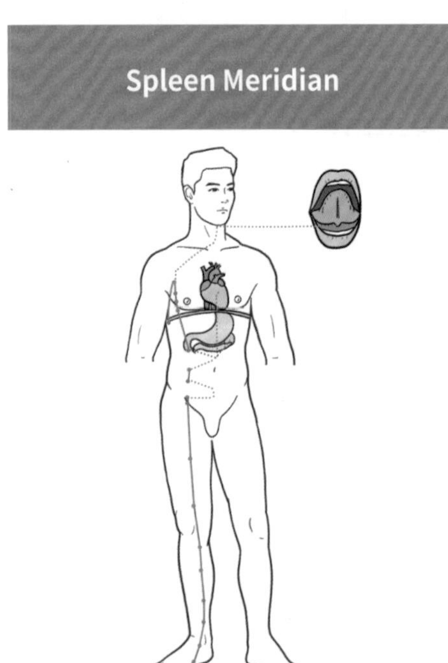

Primary Pathway

The spleen meridian begins at the big toe and runs along the inside of the foot crossing the inner ankle. It then travels along the inner side of the lower leg and thigh. Once it enters the abdominal cavity, it internally connects with the spleen and continues upward to reach the Heart Meridian. Externally, the Spleen Meridian continues moving toward the chest and branches out to reach the throat and the root of the tongue.

Main indications

Acupuncture points in this meridian are indicated for peptic, gynecological and genital diseases. They are also indicated for symptoms along the meridian.

Imbalances in the spleen meridian can be diagnosed from the mouth. Red, moist lips indicate an excess of splenetic energy while pale, dry lips indicate the opposite. A bad temper and moodiness are associated with splenetic imbalances.

Symptoms

Disharmony of the Spleen Meridian is related to spleen dysfunction.

According to TCM, the spleen is responsible for the transformation and transportation of different substances, and is the foundation of our after-birth existence. Spleen function is essential in maintaining the digestive power of the body and transforming food into qi and blood.

If the Spleen Meridian does not function properly, qi cannot be efficiently transported to the spleen.

As a result, symptoms like abdominal distention, loose stools, diarrhea, epigastric pain, flatulence and a heavy sensation in the body occur. In addition, symptoms such as pain at the root of the tongue, swelling of the inner side of the lower limb may also indicate disharmony of the Spleen Meridian.

Stiffness tongue. The early symptom of heart attack is stiff tongue. The tongue curls up and the pronunciation is unclear. The tongue is the seedling of the heart, and the spleen meridian connects to the tongue and spreads out under the tongue. Therefore, the root cause of heart disease lies in the spleen.

If the tongue is particularly flexible and soft, the person is alive, smart, reacts quickly and clever.

Puffiness tongue and tooth marks around the tongue: There is a strong stomach and weak spleen, which means that the stomach fires with strong appetite, but the spleen is weak which means unable to metabolize foods and liquid, from this, dampness is generated, and retained water and extra weight, and there are tooth marks around the tongue.

The tongue hurts, and it will immediately reflect that this is a spleen and heart disease. The spleen meridian "connects the tongue and spreads the sublingual". Spleen problems can cause Inflexible tongue movement and pain, and the tongue is the seedling of the heart, so this can also be heart blood deficiency too.

Vomiting and stomach pain. Some people vomit as soon as they eat. Stomach pain mostly relates to stomach cold.

Abdominal bloating: stomach energy goes down, spleen energy goes up, if digestion and stomach Qi cannot descend, then not only bloating, also breath will be heavy; mouthwash and freshener cannot clean the stagnate breath/ Qi in the stomach.

Another characteristic of spleen disease: feel tired after flatulence or bowel movement.

One of the characteristics of spleen disease is that the body always feels heavy. Spleen energy needs to rise, lift. If not, the person's body will become damp and heavy. Our bodies like to release it by burping and farting. That's why people burp and fart during massages.

Pain in both hips. If you want to treat spleen disease, you must first open your hips.

In Chinese medicine, diabetes is also a spleen disease, so moving the hips is to invigorate the spleen. Movement such as ballet and belly dancing, yoga, hip stretches. Diabetics usually have sweat in the upper body and no sweat in the lower body, that is, their body does not communicate up and down. If the lower body sweat can be exercised by turning the hips, the blood sugar can be normalized.

Sweating: What kind of sweating is considered good? It must be a light sweat from head to toe. Some people sweat only in the upper body, which means their body's ability to get up and down is poor. Some people only sweat on their heads, but do not sweat below their necks.

This is a yang deficiency. The heart governs the blood, and the heart is like a pump. This pump can pump blood to all the ends at once. This pump pumps on the head as well as on the feet. If your legs, feet can't sweat, even cold extremities, it's a weakness of the heart.

Muscle weakness, MS comes from spleen deficiency; unable to distribute the food essences to the limbs, the muscles will become depleted and weak. Over time, the muscles and bones are weak. Therefore, in this disease, strengthening the spleen is the first priority.

Restless leg syndrome: the cause is unknown, probably a central nervous system disorder. This kind of patient feels unbearable discomfort in the deep part of the calf when resting, which can be temporarily relieved by exercise and massage. Usually during sleep at night, extreme discomfort occurs in both lower limbs, forcing the patient to keep moving the lower limbs and walking down the ground.

In TCM theory, aging starts from the legs, and the yang qi becomes greatly deficient. In "Lingshu Tiannian," it is said that the law of yang Qi in our life is as follows:

The yang Qi of the baby is in the feet.

Before the age of 10, the yang is in the legs and feet, so children like to run and jump.

Around the age of 20, the blood is strong, the Yang Qi is in the legs, and people like to walk fast.

At the age of 30, the blood is full and the muscles are strong, so it is easy to walk.

At the age of 40, Yang Qi and blood begin to decline from the top reaching the buttocks, so like to sit.

At the age of 50, the liver Qi declines and there are diseases or problems such as eye sight weakness. Where does Yang Qi go? It goes to the back, likes to lay on the sofa, and doesn't like to sit straight anymore.

At the age of 60, the heart Qi is weak, spirit is not enough and insufficient, it is easy to be miserable. The Yang Qi is greatly weakened, like lying down.

If the Yang Qi continues to decline, the human mind will not be able to remember much.

From this point of view, the problem of the leg is Yang deficiency first; secondly, all the tremors, etc., are related to the deficiency of liver essence. At the beginning, it usually starts with shaking of the legs, which points to insufficient spleen essence and heart essence.

Acupoints

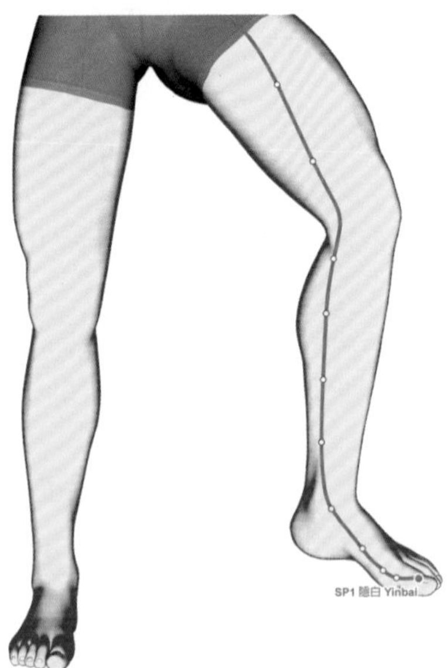

SP 1: YIN BAI (HIDDEN WHITE)

Name: Hidden White, earth is the mother of metal (Lung/L. intestine), Hidden Metal refers to phlegm that is hidden and waiting to be eliminated. Hiding from the world.

Location: 0.1 Cun posterior to the corner of the nail. On the medial side of the big toe.

Indication: Upper gastrointestinal and uterine bleeding, because "the spleen controls the blood." It can also treat acute enteritis, schizophrenia, neurasthenia, etc.

Gout: Gout usually starts at big toes. The pain is swollen and painful, and then spreads to the ankle. If the treatment is working, the pain will decrease and the pain area will shrink from ankles to toes. Then it's a good thing. When a person is old, his big toe will not be conscious, because the heart is far from the toe, and the legs and feet will get weak first.

What should I do? 1. Massage frequently, 2. Soak your feet frequently, 3. Stand on your toes then drop off heel down, this will stretch the bladder meridian. More importantly, it shakes the spine and the governor channel, moves the qi and blood flow in the meridians of the whole body. The toes are where the three yin meridians of the feet and the three yang meridians of the feet meet. Adjust the corresponding viscera function.

Mania: Mania is spleen and stomach disease, deficiency of spleen and stomach disease is depression, we have already talked about this in stomach meridian earlier. It will not be repeated here.

Techniques and notes: massage or moxibustion.

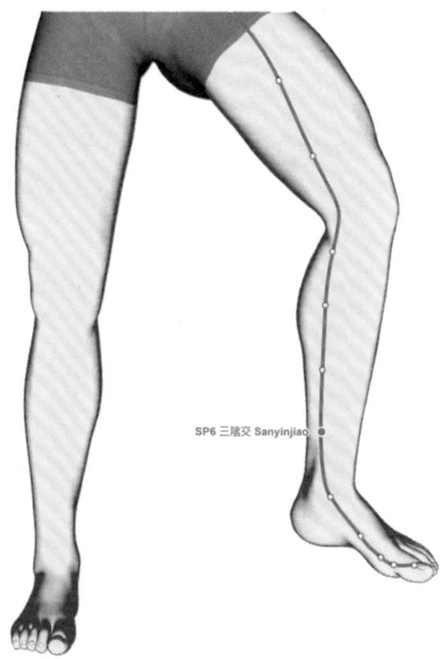

SP 6: SAN YIN JIAO (THREE YIN CROSSING)

Name: Three Yin Crossing, it refers to the intersection of the three yin meridians of the liver, spleen, and kidney, which is the fault of the three yin meridians.
Location: three Cun (three fingers) straight above the tip of the medial malleolus, at the posterior edge of the medial surface of the tibia.
Indications: stomach - spleen problem, appetite. digestion, female problems, infertility, seminal emission. urination and impotence. insomnia. high blood pressure, skin problem, irregular menstruation, uterine bleeding, leucorrhea, sterility, muscular atrophy, dizziness. Conditions of the spleen, stomach, liver and kidneys and the parts of the meridian, such as hiccups, vomiting, appetite, weakness of the spleen and stomach, fullness of the heart and abdomen, abdominal and bowel pain, edema, irregular menstruation, amenorrhea, vaginal discharge, bleeding, stillbirth, continuous lochia, penile pain and testicular pain.
Techniques and notes: massage; moxibustion can be used for 10 to 15 minutes. Can use cupping.

Because the spleen meridian is on the inner legs and thighs, it is not easy to exercise. Unlike the bladder or stomach meridian, which you can easily reach. The spleen meridian, liver meridian, and kidney must be massaged, you can lay on the bed with the bottom of your feet touching each other, and then execute opening and closing leg movements.

Massage the spleen meridian along meridian acupoints, and many body discomforts can be resolved. Relax your foot on your knee, and then use your thumbs or Gua Sha board massage along the tibia bones, from ankles to knees up to groin. In the beginning, massaging the spleen meridian can be very painful, but it will get better after a few days.

Moxibustion Zhongwan (about 4 fingers above belly button). Anyone with spleen and stomach disorders, such as hiccups, gastritis, bad breath, abdominal distension (too many people with stomach bloating now), depression, patellar softening, epilepsy, etc. can use moxa Zhongwan. *Moxibustion:* Before moxibustion, rub the Zhongwan. It is better skin flushing around and feels slightly warm. It is better to moxibustion until you sweat a little for the first time.

Miscellaneous bits

Element: Earth
Direction: Center
Season: Late Summer
Climate: Damp
Sense Organ: Mouth
Sense: Taste
Tissue: Muscles
Positive Emotion: Compassion
Negative Emotion: Anxiety
Flavor: Sweet
Color: Yellow
Sound: Singing
Smell: Fragrant
Time: 9 a.m. – 11 a.m.
Opposite: Pericardium
Yin/Yang: Yang
Flow Direction: Up
Origin/Ending: Foot to Chest
Number of Acupoints: 21 spleen meridian acupoints on one side of the body, total 42 acupoints, starting at Yinbai and ending at Dabao.

Spleen Meditation

Resting comfortably now.

Imagine now if you will, that you are standing in a garden, a garden which symbolizes your life...

And you are standing here looking around and marveling at the beauty of all the trees and the flowers and grass, in the garden of your life.

Feel the warmth of the sun shining down on you… feel a soft gentle breeze and the sweet smell of your favorite flowers. There is a mixture of annuals and perennials. Swaths of color, especially yellow, herbs, vegetables, flowers, shrubs and trees.

Notice the shrubs or bushes or other plants… maybe an jasmine-covered archway ... Notice the fertile soil. See the compost over in the corner.

Hear the birds in the trees, whistling their tunes to each other.

Imagine this… see it in your mind's eye ...

Be quiet and still. Visualize the roots of the plants plunging downward into mother earth. At the same time connecting to each other like earth meridians.

Stand in the sun and watch as the butterflies and the bees flutter around the flowers seeming to know just how to get at the sweet nectar.

Set your intention to steward over your garden. Prepare and tend to the soil. Water and feed the plants, trees and shrubs. Talk to your plants with encouragement, love and nurturing. Show your garden compassion, just as you show yourself love and compassion.

Marvel at the intelligent design, the harmony and the cooperation of flora and fauna. Rejoice in the harvest of the beautiful flowers that enrich your life and the abundance of fruits and vegetables that nourish your body and soul.

Harmonize the rhythm of your body with the garden of your life and the earth mother… vibrate as one, in sync with nature and your human nature at once and touch base with your higher self as you prepare for a journey of transformation… into the world of the spleen meridian…

Take three slow, deep breaths and prepare yourself for a meditative journey…

Take another slow deep breath… inhale and exhale…

Notice when you feel a light shift move through your entire body… the spleen Qi is about being light and uplifting…

Keep breathing, inhale and exhale…

Keep breathing and notice when you feel your body lighten, almost weightless…

And breathe, inhale and exhale…

Draw your awareness to a sense of feeling yourself getting even lighter in your body and continue breathing… inhale and exhale…

Breathing in relaxation, exhaling any tension or stress…

Notice how your understanding has expanded to see that your key to achieving your dreams and desires lies in your willingness to harmonize and balance your meridians and meridian energy, the key to knowing yourself and staying healthy, which in turn has the capacity to deliver the best you…

Become aware of the fact that you cannot control the outer world, understand that control of the outer world is an illusion ... instead, it is your inner world that you can control, and it is your meridians that connect the parts of your inner world…

Bring your awareness to learning that meditation, quiet stillness, is the gateway to "the zone"… know that mastering this recognition places you into the position that will allow you to create your reality… with practice, any mindstate can be tamed in meditation… any dream imagined and set in motion when imagined in meditation…

Give yourself permission to dive deeply into the practice of meditation… give yourself permission to believe that if you can hold it in your mind, you can hold it in your body… to recognize where you are with your meridians and no matter where that is, you can balance them through positive and loving thoughts and gentle actions…

Create an awareness of your ability to enter daily meditation for even a few minutes of quiet stillness and enter "the zone" before the avalanche of daily thoughts arrives… understand and nurture the fact that we can always, no matter the state of the world around us, bring ourselves into the zone and balance our awareness and direct our thoughts to love, kindness, gratitude and forgiveness… and beyond, to the details of our dreams…

Feel how your awareness of your meridians empowers you to alter your body's balance; how your meridian awareness can provide the opportunity to not only shift from wherever you are to balance and harmony, but also to project love and kindness to others…

Embrace the opportunity to nurture the spleen meridian, which regulates the quantity and the quality of blood in circulation and works with the lung meridian to generate true human energy ... know that this meridian is affected by the tone of your muscles and affects them in turn ... work to achieve good muscle tone and in so doing balance your spleen meridian energy… a balanced spleen meridian is responsible for logical and analytical thinking and is also the first meridian in memory formation ... understand that the spleen meridian is the gateway to mind, body and spirit…

Fully understand that with practice, meditation itself can become the venue for manifesting and the discovery and development of you ... learning to observe you and your thoughts as the first step toward moving away from powerless states of mind and a belief that external forces control you toward an empowered knowing yourself state.…

Visualize yourself engaged in this daily personal meditative practice as not just an inoculation against imbalanced meridians and deficient Qi, but the avenue to meridian balance and harmony through the act of intention and living an intentional life…

See yourself grounded, balanced and clear on your growing ability to balance your meridians… see the mastery of your yin/yang balance being the foundation for the ability to bring your self-awareness to who you are and who you want to be regardless of where you may have started from ... and from there, deliberately achieving optimal health…

Understand that balancing your meridians is the key to health, wealth and happiness ... when we are balanced and in harmony, we engage the universe in giving us what we want…

Give yourself permission to practice resting in an energetic field of pure potential… mastering meditation, building strength of mind and developing the skill of balancing your meridians on demand...

Understand that meditation is your pathway to cultivate your greatest balance and harmony… your lightest and most uplifting actions and goals… it is through this balance and harmony that we can also nurture love, kindness, and forgiveness for self and others.…

Continue beyond and see that beginning your day in the meditation zone and balancing your Qi will begin to allow you to alter and influence the outer world, while also understanding illusion and that you will never "control" it...

Feel the satisfaction of allowing the power of balance and harmony with your meridians to help you live a healthy life, being in flow, and recognizing the power of surrender and the magic that comes from setting it and allowing it to happen...

Know that the spleen meridian begins at the big toe and runs along the inside of the foot crossing the inner ankle. It then travels along the inner side of the lower leg and thigh. Once it enters the abdominal cavity, it internally connects with the spleen and continues upward to reach the Heart Meridian. Externally, the Spleen Meridian continues moving toward the chest and branches out to reach the throat and the root of the tongue.

Breathe in these changes as you understand that they will not come overnight, but will be molded over a course of ongoing experiences and learnings… know that these experiences and learnings will help you create and define your inner world ...

Know that the spleen meridian includes the pancreas and is involved in digestion… The spleen is referred to as the "Minister of the Granary." Nutrients from food and beverages are extracted by enzymes produced in the spleen and pancreas.

The spleen meridian regulates the quantity and the quality of blood in circulation and works with the lung meridian to generate True Human Energy… This meridian is affected by the tone of muscles and affects them in turn. The spleen meridian is responsible for logical and analytical thinking. It is also the first meridian in memory formation…

Embrace that it is meditation and the meditative attitude that will plant the seed and accelerate your growth… that you will reap immeasurable blessings through your spiritual journey ... be prepared for your life to continue to undergo positive transformations as you learn more about the meridians and yourself every day ... understand that you will be able to fulfill your worldly duties and desires, while building a stronger connection within your own meridian system and with the universe beyond ...

Begin to foresee the power of harmonious meridians... and breathe...

Notice the vibration now that is building stronger and stronger and stronger still in your body and notice how strength of mind is washing over you...

Bring your awareness to the breath and the body as a whole, breathing and resting here for this period of time, enjoy this relatively stable platform of moment-to-moment awareness, riding on the waves of the breath....

Set your intention to grow awareness of your power of meridian balance and harmony and understand that you can resist riding the stream like a helpless leaf, resist blaming external forces for anything in your life, instead shaping your experience by setting your intention to achieve what you want and thereby affect your outer world experience...

Prepare for making the unconscious conscious through meditation, which will result in balanced meridians, enhanced focus, increased emotional intelligence, greater mental strength, improved physical health, healthy relationships, lasting, holistic happiness and ultimately to self-realization...

Internalize the idea that YOU matter, and that there is a hidden purpose and reason for who you are and where you are in life... AND with hard work, you can find it.... AND that as you find yourself you will be in a better position to lift others...

Notice the sensations and breathe... inhale and exhale...

Understand that you and your meridians are far more interesting than any low vibrational events currently circulating on the news or masquerading as entertainment... and as you do, your thoughts will become filled with meaning the moment you think they are... And meditation is the pathway to creating balance and creating you....

Give yourself permission for a new awareness of your power to create reality through the balancing of your meridians, through meditation and how this awareness will prepare you to live fully and healthily…

Bring your awareness to the smile on your face as you realize that the privilege of a lifetime is to become who you truly are and that becoming permeates your body, mind and soul…

Now that you are coming through all of this, notice the happiness you feel inside knowing how powerful meridian balance is and how connected to humanity you are…notice how this connection fills you with an elevated vibration… and how much YOU you feel…

Now just breathe and be with yourself and let the waves of your breathing be with you…

CHAPTER FIVE

Heart Meridian

Characteristics

The heart has two characteristics, one is that the heart controls the blood vessels, and the other is that the heart controls the spirits.

The "King of the Organs," the heart is the house of the vital essence. It commands all of the other organs and emotions. The heart is also seen as the seat of the mind. It works with many organs to regulate circulation and maintain a healthy mental state. If the heart is imbalanced, all the other organs and meridians will suffer. It is also seen as primary in the defense against disease.

Before we dive into the heart meridian, let's understand the meridian flow, each meridian works for two hours, so total 12 meridians cover 24 hours a day.

From 11 am to 1 pm, meridian Qi mainly flows through the Heart meridian, this is the best time to have conversations and connect with people. Reach out to people, cooperate, be of service.

Eat a nutritious, balanced lunch, but not too filling (eating too much at lunch will make you want to nap!).

Heart Meridian

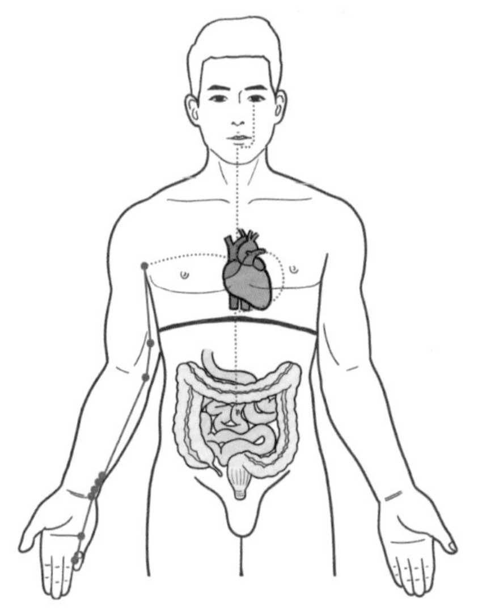

Primary Pathway

The Heart Meridian starts from the heart and divides into three branches. One branch goes towards the small intestine. The second branch runs upwards along the throat towards the eyes, and the third branch emerges under the arm and runs along the inner side of the forearm, elbow and upper arm; it then crosses the inner side of the wrist and palm and ends at the inside tip of the little finger, where it connects with the small intestine meridian.

The spleen meridian ends at the heart, the spleen meridian and the heart meridian are connected. When a heart attack occurs, the tongue feels tight. In fact, it is also connected to the chin. When a person is angry, the chin shakes, which means that the heart is throbbing, and it is difficult for the person to speak. Generally speaking, people with big chins are calm, people with small chins are smart but a little short-tempered. As for officials and business people, most of them have big chins. Such people have strong heart energy and resist oppression.

The heart belongs to the Shaoyin of the hand, and the kidney belongs to the Shaoyin of the foot. Both of them are power sources in our human body and are the most powerful among the organs.

Heart and kidney are the two most important things in our life. The power of life is strong, and it belongs to the heart and kidneys; if our body is to be able to transform and create life, it is also a matter of the heart and the kidneys.

In TCM the heart meridian is not only the heart organ, but a system called the "heart system."

This heart system includes the heart organ, heart meridian, heart governing the blood vessels, the heart governing the spirits, the heart serving as the official of the monarch, etc. It also includes the liver wood generating the heart fire, the heart fire generating the spleen earth, and the heart fire controlling the lung metal, these are all in the same system, all on the same team, and they all affect the whole body.

Therefore, Chinese medicine looks at any organ from the perspective of the system, not from the organ.

So, in TCM the "heart" has at least three levels. First, the heart organ, which is what western medicine refers to. Second, heart Qi, refers to the heart meridian; heart governs blood vessels, the heart and small intestine are external and internal, the heart opens up in both ears and the heart is in the will and joy. Third, the seat of the mind and spirit, that is, the heart controls the spirit of the mind.

For example, the function of the heart that governs blood is Qi level. Cold hands and feet mean a weak function of the heart governing the blood vessels, that is, the heart cannot pump blood to the extremities of the hands and feet. The hands and feet are the places you can touch, but did you know that the top of the head and the uterus belong to the extremities, too? It follows then, that people with cold hands and feet also can have a cold uterus as well as memory loss and mental decline.

In short, every organ has three levels: shape, Qi, and Shen. Shape, refers to organs; Qi, refers to meridians; Shen, refers to spirit. Western medicine generally only pays attention to the aspect of shape, and the aspects of Qi and spirit are still the most talked about in TCM. At the level of Qi, Chinese medicine has the theory of meridians, and at the level of Shen or spirit, TCM has the theory of Five Organs in relationship with emotion and spirits. Starting from the meridians, it is easiest to understand the Qi in Chinese medicine.

The heart meridian starts from the heart, and divides into three branches. One goes towards the small intestine.

The heart and the small intestine are in the same family, husband and wife, one is outside and the other is inside. When the heart is unhappy, a bad mood will sink to the bottom, the small intestine will be sad too. This will lead to the small intestine unable to absorb nutrients. Long-term nutritional deficiencies will make people empty. Any intestinal cancer, doesn't matter if its large intestine or small intestine cancer can be linked to many years of unhappiness! But few doctors see this level.

The second runs upwards along the throat towards the eyes.

'Ihe third branch emerges under thc arm and runs along the inner side of the forearm, commonly known as the "butterfly sleeve" place.

Main Indication

Acupuncture points in this meridian are indicated for heart, chest and mental problems. They are also indicated for symptoms along the meridian.

Symptoms

Problems in the nose and throat are related to extreme thinking and anxiety, and extreme thinking must contain the extremes of human nature. The extreme of human nature relates to extreme ego. This extreme self will definitely imprint on one's life, and this imprint leads to disease.

Colon cancer and nasopharyngeal carcinoma are two different diseases on the surface, but they are actually one disease. The human body is the cavity, the nasopharynx is the upper opening, and the large intestine is the lower opening. If the upper opening is blocked, the lower opening must be blocked; if the lower opening is blocked, the upper opening will not be cured. It's just that the nasopharynx is directly connected to the brain, so it is much more problematic than the lower opening.

Eye disease is also a big problem in modern times.

The visual function of the eyes is mainly controlled by the heart, this is because the heart masters the spirit. Eye is the window of the spirit. The excessive use of the eyes now leads to dry eyes, blurred vision, high eye pressure, floaters, etc., and are also related to liver blood deficiency.

There are four simple ways to protect the eyes:

Warm the eyes with palms. Quickly rub the palms until warm, then cover eyes with both palms. Do this 36 times per day.

Massage the "rear eye point" on the back of the head (there are two small dents on the back of the head opposite the eyes, and the area with high eye pressure will bulge.

Circle your eyes in four directions: up, left, down then right. Repeat 36 times or more.

Life is diminished by overuse. Don't stay up late, don't bring your mobile phone into the bedroom, spend less time on your phone. This is the best way to nourish your eyes.

As we age, especially women, tend to have loose upper arms, called "butterfly sleeves ". In fact, this is the result of heart Qi, small intestine and spleen energy weak and deficient.

When people are older and can still can wear sleeveless dresses or clothes that are tight around the arm muscles display signs of good health. So, what can we do? Grab, rub and massage this place frequently, or grab a water bottle with both hands and raise it above your head, and tap your upper back, not only to exercise your arms, but also to prevent the effects of aging.

Disharmony of the heart meridian leads to pain at the heart position (pericardial pain or pain at the sternum).

In TCM, the heart rules the blood and the pulse. Without sufficient nourishment, an individual may have following symptoms:

Thirst and dry throat. When we are in a hurry, our throat will immediately become hot and dry, and we may not even be able to swallow.

Heartache, heavy breath, sudden stiffness of the tongue, etc., all demonstrate the risk of heart disease.

There are a few reasons for heart pain in TCM, pain due to myocardial ischemia, pain due to obstruction, or stasis of meridians, pain due to lack of heart Yang, pain due to water and damp stasis.

Dizziness, vomiting, sweating, feeling unhappy, etc. This is very similar to the early stage of myocardial infarction.

Pain in the inner side of the forearm or the arm is sore and weak.

For example, before a heart attack, there may be a pain in the shoulder and back, and the pain can radiate to one or both arms, shoulders, wrists, fingers, and upper back.

Arm muscle weakness or numbness and pain are the lack of heart Qi. In the early stages of heart disease, pain in the upper part of the arm occurs. Often massaging or slapping here will have a very good preventive effect.

Brain problems, memory loss, confusion, forgetfulness, etc.

How does the heart relate to the brain? The heart meridian does not travel to the head. Wood generates fire, liver and gallbladder are wood elements, and heart is fire element, that is, the liver and gallbladder meridians go to the head, and the heart blood is carried from the liver and gallbladder to the head.

Clear mind is associated with the liver and gallbladder. If the liver and gallbladder are overactive and take too much blood to the brain, the blood pressure is high. Why does the liver and gallbladder have no restraints and overreact? The problem lies in the kidneys.

The kidneys are water, so they can't be pulled from underneath, they go up. When the kidney water also declines, it means that the pressure is high, and it starts to consume the old money (our reserve), which is the kidney.

As a result, diastolic pressure is high, also called renal hypertension. Systolic blood pressure is a sign that the heart and liver are still strong, while diastolic pressure is high and the kidney is weak.

Hot and pain in the palm. There are two diseases in the palm, one is heat and the other is pain.

If there is a heart problem, it will be dry and itchy at the interface of the little finger, hypothenar area.

Acupoints

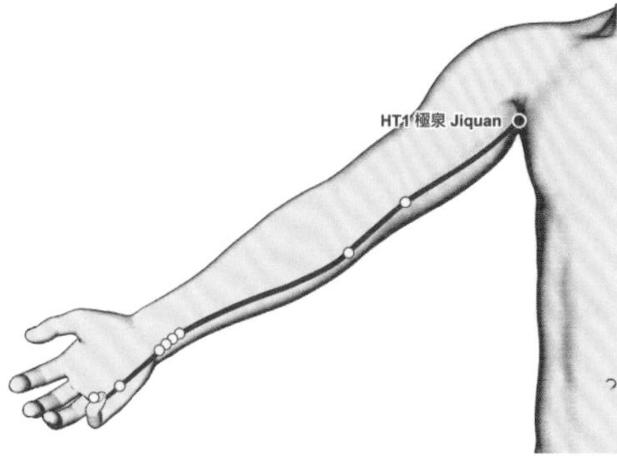

HT 1: JI QUAN (UTMOST SPRING)

Name: Utmost Spring, the Heart begins with the spring of endless possibilities. It helps connect to spirit. Connecting to the sources of the Utmost Love, it's not the highest point on the physical body, but it reaches the highest level. Rubbing the Jiquan Point can make you happy.

Location: With the upper arm abducted, the point is in the center of the axilla, medial to the axillary artery. The method of taking Jiquan point, abduct the upper arm, at the apex of the axilla, where the axillary artery pulses.

Indication: Many women's Jiquan acupoint is particularly painful, which is related to long-term emotional discomfort.

Heartache, palpitations. Chest tightness, shortness of breath, and flank pain. Shoulder and arm pain, upper limb paralysis, scrofula, etc.

Techniques and notes: Rub and massage.

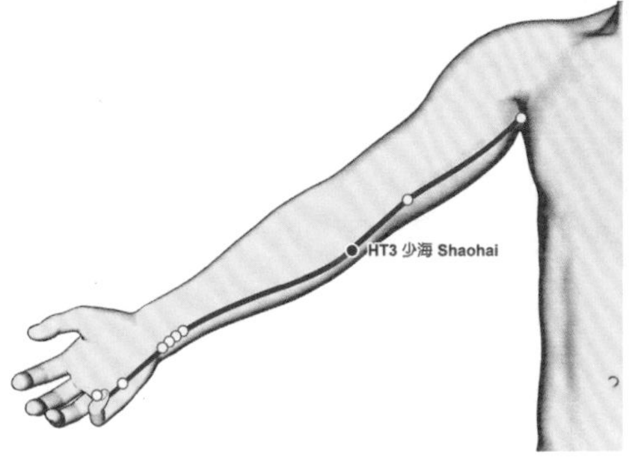

HT 3: SHAO HAI (LESSER SEA)

Name: Shao Hai, Shao, refers to the Shaoyin heart meridian; the sea is the confluence of all rivers, and it is infinitely deep and wide. The Chinese character "Sea " is the image of a woman lying on the seashore, which means that the sea is like a mother and is the source of life, so any acupuncture point called the "sea" are all rooted things and cannot be ignored.

Location: bend the elbow, at the depression of the ulnar crease of the cubital crease. Between the medial end of the transverse cubital crease and the medial epicondyle of the tumorous.

Indication: treats diseases of the seven emotions, such as madness, drooling, and neck pain, arm pain, toothache, dizziness and so on.

Techniques and notes: Rub and massage.

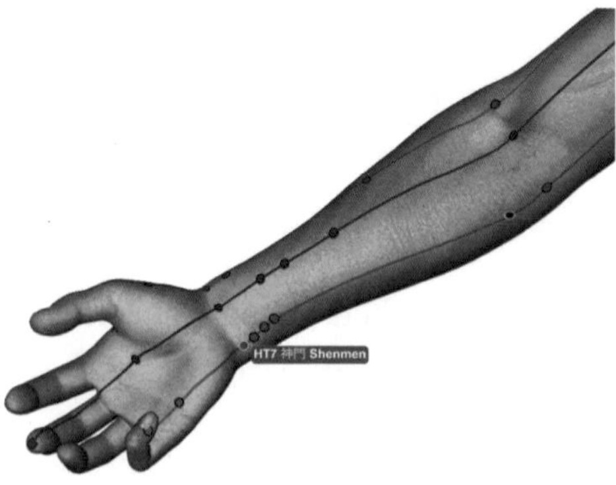

HT 7: SHEN MEN (SPIRIT'S GATE)

Name: Spirit's gate, where the spirits enter and exit.

Location: Go up along the red and white flesh marks of the arm to the depression on the radial side of the transverse wrist crease. There is an acupuncture point called Shenmen.

Indication: heart pain, chest pain, heartache, upset, palpitations, forgetfulness, insomnia, dementia, epilepsy, motion sickness, high blood pressure.

Techniques and notes: It is best to pinch, rub, and press this point before going to bed.

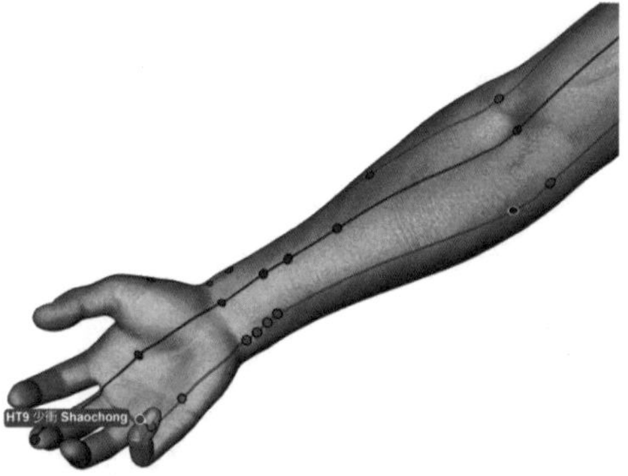

HT 9: SHAO CHONG (LESSER SURGE)

Name: Lesser Surge, not that there is freedom - you do not need another incarnation - your Chong is fulfilled.

Location: 0.1 cun posterior to the corner of the nail, on the radial side of the little finger.

Indication: mainly treats palpitations, heartache, chest pain, mania, fever, coma, hand spasm and arm pain. The tingling of the little finger is definitely related to the heart.

Techniques and notes: massage your tip of ten fingers off and on, it will definitely be beneficial to the internal organs.

How to nourish the heart?

Talk less. Words are the voice of the heart. Talking too much can consume energy and effort, so lecturing is not only a mental task, but also a laborious task. Moreover, interpersonal communication should be more and more refined, less socializing, and no debate or quarrel when it comes to matters of the heart.

Don't take everything too seriously.

Don't sweat profusely. It is normal to sweat in summer, but if you sweat profusely during exercise too often, or have abnormal sweat all year round, like hot flashes and cold flashes, you should be careful, because sweat is the liquids of the heart, and if you sweat too much, you will deplete your heart Qi and blood. It is best to find a good doctor and get treated, don't let it go.

The most important function of the heart is to "govern the internal organs," that is to say, everything in the body is under the control of the heart, not specifically to manage, but to control.

This is also emphasizing the power of the heart. With this power of the heart Qi, the internal organs will not dare to mess around. On the other hand, if one's heart Qi is off balance, the internal organs will be in chaos.

A good life needs a good mood. But when people get sick, they never think about their emotions, they just look for various external causes. This is the foolishness and sadness of human beings.

One of the benefits of learning the meridians and acupoints is that you can figure out which meridian might have a problem from where there is pain and discomfort or skin irritations, etc.

For example, if you have pain in your arm or elbow, you just need to remember that there are three Yin meridians inside of the arm: the lung meridian, the pericardium meridian, and the heart meridian, and three Yang meridians are top and outside of the arm: Large Intestine, Sanjiao, and Small Intestine.

From there you should carefully distinguish whether pain is near the inside of the elbow or arm which is close to heart meridian or outer arm close to large intestine meridian or lung meridian.

The human body has its own big medicine, and the big medicine is the meridians and acupuncture points.

Miscellaneous bits:

Element: Fire
Direction: South
Season: Summer
Climate: Heat
Sense Organ: Tongue
Sense: Touch
Tissue: Vessels
Positive Emotion: Joy
Negative Emotion: Arrogance
Flavor: Bitter
Color: Red
Sound: Laughter
Smell: Scorched
Time: 11 a.m. - 1 p.m.
Opposite: Gall Bladder
Yin/Yang: Yin
Flow Direction: Up
Origin/Ending: Chest to Hand
Number of Acupoints: 9 on one side of the body, total 18 on both side of the body.

Heart Meditation

Resting comfortably now.

Begin by sitting in a comfortable position and close your eyes.

For just this moment, let go of your thoughts and the outside world.

Focus your attention on your spiritual heart center, in the middle of your chest, and be aware of your heart as a space ... The heart center is a point of awareness where feelings enter ... let's begin a sacred journey…

At its essence, the heart is pure emptiness, pervaded by peace and a subtle light ... This light may appear as white, gold, pale pink, or green ... But don't strain to find a light of any kind ... All you need to feel is whatever is there ....

In your imagination, I'd like you to take yourself to a beautiful place in nature. Perhaps on a peaceful island or maybe out in the country or maybe a mountain trail - your perfect setting. Create a wonderful day - a warm, summer afternoon or early evening - a soft, gentle breeze that gently caresses your skin and your hair - and there's nothing that you need to do right now, just enjoy your special place.

Imagine yourself resting, perhaps on a tree stump, or a cluster of rocks - watching your perfect scene. The sun is beginning to set and you watch as it gradually lowers over the horizon - covering the once blue sky with beautiful splashes of color - crimson streaks and yellow-gold - blends into the endless blue - as you sit and watch.

And before your eyes, the colors and hues begin to change as the sky becomes darker - appears like a slender giant with a purple robe, languishing lazily, drifting - and your mind may begin to drift a little as you go deeper into trance - that wonderful, comfortable state of relaxation deep within you.

And enjoy your perfect place. Let the colors of the sunset fill the space in your inner mind, and the colors may change from time to time as the sun goes down and darkness falls.

Imagine a curtain - a veil or a cloak being drawn across the sunset of your mind. And the colors are still there, on the other side of the cloak but now all that you see is darkness - darkness in place of color - but it's a comfortable darkness - it's safe - secure - like strong arms wrapped around a newborn baby that snuggles down into comfortable repose after all of its physical and spiritual needs have been met.

You can feel yourself drifting down deeper, deeper within yourself, falling, descending - deeper and deeper relaxed.

It is a comfortable feeling here. There is a peaceful serenity deep within you, it makes you feel calm, it makes you feel relaxed - calm, relaxed and confident, calm, comfortable and so relaxed.

Just allow yourself to feel joy.

Be quiet and still. Visualize putting roots downward into mother earth. Ground yourself like earthbound meridians.

Set your intention to live in balance. Show yourself love and compassion, just as you show others love and compassion.

Bringing your attention back gently… easily… to your heart center… breathe gently and sense your breath flowing into your heart ... You may want to visualize a soft, pastel light or coolness permeating the chest ...

Let your breath go in and out, and as it does, ask your heart what it needs to say ... Don't phrase this as an order… just have the indistinct intention that you want your heart to express itself...

Listen to your heart… Your heart will begin to release emotions, memories, wishes, fears, and dreams long stored inside ... just be quiet and still and listen… As your heart releases, allow yourself to pay attention ...

You may have a flash of strong emotions… could be positive or negative… or perhaps a forgotten memory ... You may find your breathing change ... You may gasp, sigh, or feel tears come into your eyes ... if so, continue to allow and accept… Let the experience be what it is…

If you daydream or drift off into what feels like sleep, don't worry… Just bring your attention back to your heart center...

Vow to talk less ... understand that words are the voice of the heart ... talking too much can consume energy and effort… know that lecturing is not only a mental task, but also a laborious task ... know that interpersonal communication should be more and more refined… less socializing… and no debate or quarrel when it comes to matters of the heart...

Don't take everything too seriously.

Be careful not to sweat profusely… It is normal to sweat in summer, but if you sweat profusely during exercise too much, or have abnormal sweat all year round, like hot flashes and cold flashes, you should be careful… because sweat is the liquids of the heart…, and if you sweat too much, you will deplete your heart Qi and blood…

Take three slow, deep breaths and embrace the power of this meditative journey…

Take another slow deep breathe… inhale and exhale…

Breathing in relaxation, exhaling any tension or stress…

Notice how your understanding has expanded to see that your key to achieving your dreams and desires lies in your willingness to harmonize and balance your meridians and meridian energy, the key to knowing yourself and staying healthy, which in turn has the capacity to deliver the best you…

Resist the age old temptation to control the outer world… understand that control of the outer world is an illusion ... instead, it is your inner world that you can control, and it is your meridians that connect the parts of your inner world…

Bring your awareness to learning that meditation, quiet stillness, is the gateway to "the zone"… know that mastering this recognition places you into the position that will allow you to create your reality… with practice, any mindstate can be tamed in meditation… any dream imagined and set in motion when imagined in meditation…

Feel how your awareness of your meridians empowers you to alter your body's balance; how your meridian awareness can provide the opportunity to not only shift from wherever you are to balance and harmony, but also to project love and kindness to others…

Understand that the heart meridian starts from the heart and divides into three branches... One branch goes towards the small intestine... The second branch runs upwards along the throat towards the eyes… and the third branch emerges under the arm and runs along the inner side of the forearm, elbow and upper arm; it then crosses the inner side of the wrist and palm and ends at the inside tip of the little finger, where it connects with the small intestine meridian.

Embrace the opportunity to nurture the heart meridian… know that the heart is the King of the Organs… the heart is the house of the vital essence ... accept that the heart commands all of the other organs and emotions ... The heart is also seen as the seat of the mind ... It works with many organs to regulate circulation and maintain a healthy mental state ... If the heart is imbalanced, all the other organs and meridians will suffer ... know that the heart is also seen as primary in the defense against disease…

Fully understand that with practice, meditation itself can become the venue for manifesting and the discovery and development of you ... learning to observe yourself and your thoughts can be the first step toward moving away from powerless states of mind and a belief that external forces control you toward an empowered state of knowing yourself…

Visualize yourself engaged in this daily personal meditative practice as a guard against imbalanced meridians and deficient Qi… know that meditation can be your pathway to meridian balance and harmony through the act of intention and living an intentional life…

See yourself grounded, balanced and clear on your growing ability to balance your meridians… see the mastery of your yin/yang balance being the foundation for the ability to bring your self-awareness to who you are and who you want to be regardless of where you may have started from ... and from there, deliberately achieving optimal health…

Give yourself permission to practice resting in an energetic field of pure potential… mastering meditation, building strength of mind and developing the skill of balancing your meridians on demand...

Feel the satisfaction of allowing the power of balance and harmony with your meridians to help you live a healthy life, being in flow, and recognizing the power of surrender and the magic that comes from setting it and allowing it to happen...

Begin to foresee the power of harmonious meridians… and breathe…

Notice the vibration now that is building stronger and stronger and stronger still in your body and notice how strength of mind is washing over you…

Bring your awareness to the breath and the body as a whole, breathing and resting here for this period of time, enjoy this relatively stable platform of moment-to-moment awareness, riding on the waves of the breath....

Set your intention to grow awareness of your power of meridian balance and harmony and understand that you can resist riding the stream like a helpless leaf, resist blaming external forces for anything in your life, instead shaping your experience by setting your intention to achieve what you want and thereby affect your outer world experience...

Draw your attention to the warmth in your heart now... like a wave cresting, a wave of inner awareness, notice how it feels to be drawn into that wave... feel a sense of your increased knowing transmuting into warmth to a dozen others...

Bring your awareness to the smile on your face as you realize that the privilege of a lifetime is to become who you truly are and that becoming permeates your body, mind and soul...

Now that you are coming through all of this, notice the happiness you feel inside knowing how powerful meridian balance is and how connected to humanity you are...notice how this connection fills you with an elevated vibration... and how much YOU feel...

Now just breathe and be with yourself and let the waves of your breathing be with you...

CHAPTER SIX

Small Intestine Meridian

Characteristics

The small intestine meridian is responsible for receiving food during the digestion process. The small intestine is known as the "Minister of Reception." It separates impurities from the food before passing the waste on and also absorbs water.

One of the functions of the small intestine is the main absorption, kind of like the IRS, collecting the money and absorbing the essence. It collects a lot of good things, but it can't use it by itself. It must take out its essence and turn it over to the "treasury," and then Yuanqi, prenatal Qi will be the administrator and expenditure officer of the treasury.

From one pm to three pm, meridian Qi mainly flows through the small intestine meridian. This is the best time to solve your problems and get organized. Sort out issues. The body is digesting lunch.

Anatomically speaking, the small intestine is located in the abdomen, the upper end is connected with the pylorus and the stomach, and the lower end is connected with the large intestine through the appendix door.

This is the main location for food digestion and absorption. The small intestine is coiled in the abdominal cavity, connected to the stomach pylorus above, and the cecum below, with a total length of about four to six meters, and is divided into three parts: duodenum, jejunum and ileum. After the chemical digestion of the pancreatic enzyme, bile and small intestinal enzyme in the small intestine and the mechanical digestion of the small intestinal movement, the digestion process is basically completed, and the nutrients are absorbed by the small intestinal mucosa. It is to transform the digestible part of food into the most basic and simple element that the human body can absorb - essence.

Small Intestine Meridian

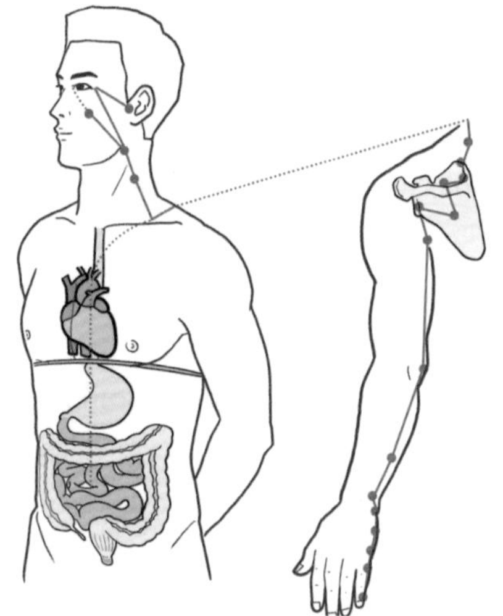

Primary Pathway

The small intestine meridian starts from the tip of the little finger and crosses the palm and wrist.

It runs upwards along the posterior side of the forearm until it reaches the back of the shoulder where it ends at the uppermost part of the back (the bottom of the neck).

At this position, it first branches off and moves internally through the heart and stomach to reach the small intestine.

The second branch travels externally across the neck and cheek until it reaches the outer corner of the eye and then enters the ear.

A short branch in the cheek moves upward to the inner corner of the eye where it connects with the bladder meridian.

At the bottom of the neck the meridian enters an area known as the "Empty Basin" (top of shoulder area). It first branches off and moves internally through the heart and stomach to reach the small intestine.

When entering the Empty Basin, everyone must remember that all the Yang meridians enter here to internal organs, such as the stomach and small intestine meridians, Triple Warmer meridian and large intestine meridian, so the Empty Basin is a key point. It can be said that it is the death point of the human body, because the Empty Basin directly leads to the internal organs. The way to protect here is to use the palm to cover the top of the shoulder, and press and knead slowly. Wearing a scarf at winter time is not only to protect the neck from the cold, but also to protect the Empty Basin.

The heart and the small intestine are in the same family, internal and external, and the nutrition of the small intestine is also perfused into the heart.

The second branch travels externally across the neck and cheek until it reaches the outer corner of the eye and then enters the ear.

Deafness and tinnitus are related to the Yang deficiency in the small intestine, the heart and the small intestine are external and internal, so sadness can lead to tinnitus; the Triple Warmer and gallbladder meridian also travel to the ear.

A short branch in the cheek moves upward to the inner corner of the eye where it connects with the bladder meridian.

This branch from the cheek goes through the eye bags area to the inner corner of the eye.

Which meridians are related to eye bags? Gallbladder, small intestine and Triple Warmer meridians. It can be seen that the essence of eye bags is Yang deficiency and cannot metabolize water. Why do you not have eye bags when you are young? Yang Qi is usually strong in youth. If you have eye bags when you are old it is usually an indication that Yang Qi is weak. Treating eye bags is accomplished by improving and raising Yang Qi. Scraping around eyes with a jade Guasha board, moxibustion using Zhongwan, Guanyuan, and herb medicines for raising Yang, this is a very good way to reduce eye bags.

How to use a Jade board to facial Gua Sha?

1. Scrape from the chin to the ears on both sides, which can lift the face and prevent aging.
2. Scrape from the Yingxiang point, next to the nose to the temple, you can lift the facial muscles, because the deep nasolabial folds will make you look old.
3. Scarp from eye bags to temple, will reduce eye bags and wrinkles around eyes.

4. Scrape the Yintang part between the two eyebrows. In this place, there is nothing to feel when you press or rub it with your finger, but when you scrape it, you feel that there are many bumps inside. It can be seen that we have worries on our brows.

The small intestine relates to nutrition. Someone with an over-nourished small intestine will have a double chin.

However, if there is over nutrition with a cold small intestine, the chin area will have acne, black heads and appear thick and oily. This is related to the lack of Yang Qi.

Young people usually have acne around the cheek, forehead. Older people usually have acne on the chin area.

Responsible for receiving and transforming food during the digestion process, the small intestine as we know is known as the "Minister of Reception." It separates impurities from the food before passing the waste on and also absorbs water.

Main indications

Acupuncture points in this meridian are indicated for diseases of the head, neck, ears, eyes and pharynx (throat), as well as certain febrile conditions and mental illnesses. These acupuncture points are also recommended for symptoms associated with the meridian's pathway.

Separating fluids, clearing and secreting turbidity of body liquids, the small intestine is responsible for body fluid problems. Here, it has two meanings: one is conditions of body fluids; second, refers to small intestine management of the distribution of the body fluids in the body.

The normal state of body fluids are: liver fluid is tears, kidney fluid is saliva, spleen fluid is mucus, heart fluid is sweat, and lung fluid is phlegm.

There are five kinds of abnormal states of body fluids: 1) In the cold weather, we urinate more frequently and we can see our breath when we exhale; 2) In hot weather, we sweat more; 3) Tears come with sadness and anger; 4) When the spleen and stomach are weak, it is manifested as mucus;

5) When the meridian Qi is blocked and the blood stagnates, it will be manifested as water swelling.

Mental clarity and discernment: the small intestine works with the heart meridian. It controls the basic emotions and the Chinese equivalent of "a broken heart" is "broken intestines." The meridian also works with the pituitary gland, also known as the "master gland," to regulate growth and the endocrine system.

The judgment and decision making is dependent on the heart being strong. Heart fire can be transferred to small intestines.

Imbalance in the small intestine meridian can cause emaciation and pain in the abdomen. It can also lead to poor reasoning ability and restlessness.

The heart is determined to be happy, if the person is not happy, the pain will sink to the bottom and affect the small intestine. No matter if one has colorectal cancer or small intestinal cancer, there is definitely one reason for it, they have been unhappy for years, but few doctors see or understand at this level.

Symptoms

Disharmony of the small intestine meridian presents mainly as symptoms along its pathway such as:

Swollen cheeks or bags under the eyes. The small intestine channel "does not cross the cheeks," that is, from the cheeks to the bags under the eyes, this area is swollen, and it is also a manifestation of the deficiency of the Yang Qi of the small intestine channel.

Neck, jaw, shoulder, elbow, arm pain, along the small intestine line. The small intestine meridian cannot get cold, but the small intestine meridian is the most susceptible to cold. If you suffer from a cold in the shoulders and neck, the most effective ones are moxibustion and cupping. Massage is not easy to drive out the cold energy, unless you sweat while massaging, then wipe the sweat off, and don't get caught in the wind.

Deafness is one of the main symptoms of the small intestine meridian because the small intestine meridian traverses the neck and upper cheeks to the eye and canthus (the outer or inner corner of the eye, where the upper and lower lids meet), then enters the ear. If the small intestine gets cold and you are anxious, it can directly cause deafness. In comparison, sudden deafness is easier to treat than tinnitus, because sudden deafness is an acute disease, while tinnitus is a chronic disease. However, if the elderly gradually become deaf, it is due to the loss of kidney essence, and the sea of marrow is empty. The treatment will be slower.

Tinnitus: of the six Yang meridians, only the large intestine meridian does not travel to the ear. The rest of the meridians all travel through the ear. Therefore, tinnitus is a deficiency of Yang Qi. Excessive depression or exposure to cold can also cause tinnitus. In spring, there are still many people feeling pressure and fullness on the ears, and the inside has a feeling of collapse or tiredness. That's deficit of vital Qi, this condition prevents distribution of Qi to the rest of the body. It's difficult to treat deafness and tinnitus in both TCM and western medicine.

Yellow eyes. The small intestine meridian runs from the empty basin to the upper cheeks of the neck, to the inner side of the eyes. That is, the inner and outer corners of the eyes belong to the small intestine meridian. If the small intestine meridian of the Yang energy is insufficient, the eyes will be yellow.

Acupoints

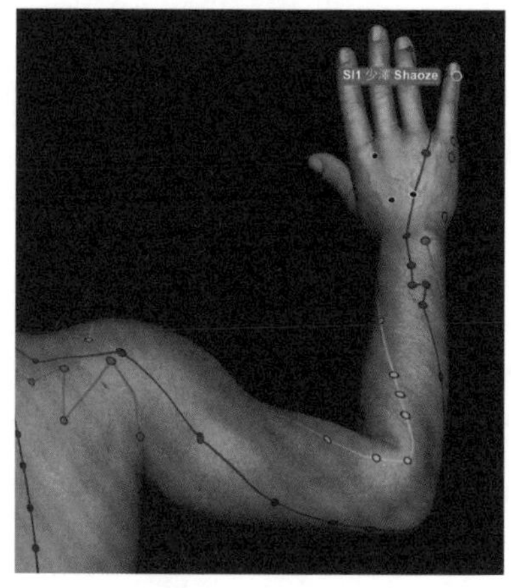

SI 1 SHAO ZE (LESSER MARSH)

Name: Lesser Marsh, Marsh is a place where people hide. This is a place of latency. It helps to draw out that which is latent. Bring someone out of a state of confusion, daydreaming, stupor.

Location: 0.1 cun posterior to the corner of the nail, on the ulnar aspect of the little finger.

Connected with the Heart meridian, the Heart meridian "goes out from the inside of the little finger", which is the relationship between the heart and the small intestine.

Indication:

1. Lack of breast milk, it is mainly used for breast diseases such as breast carbuncle and lack of milk. The ten fingertips can be used to massage the fingertips with the thumb and index finger.
2. Fainting, coma, fever and other emergencies, heat syndrome,
3. Five sense diseases such as sore throat, headache, blurred vision.. But not for pregnant women.

Techniques and notes: massage.

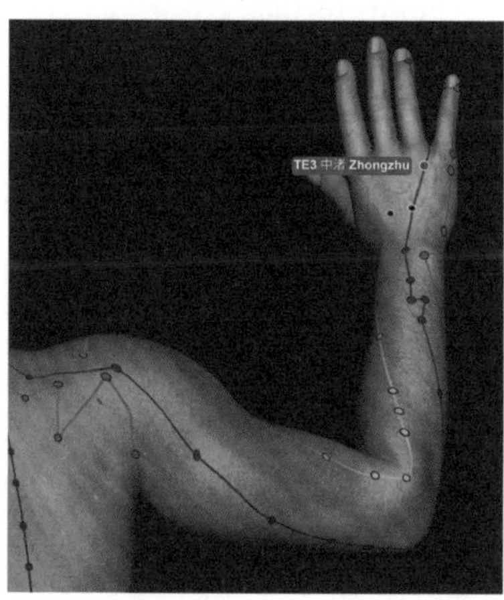

SI 3 HOU XI (BLACK RAVINE)

Name: Behind the ravine - back and bladder

Location: On the ulnar side of hand, proximal to the fifth metacarpophalangeal joint, at the end of the transverse crease and the border of the dark and light skin

Indication:

1. Eyes, ear and throat problem
2. Back pain, stiff neck
3. Mental issues.
4. Regulates sweeting
5. Urine problems.

Techniques and notes: Massage.

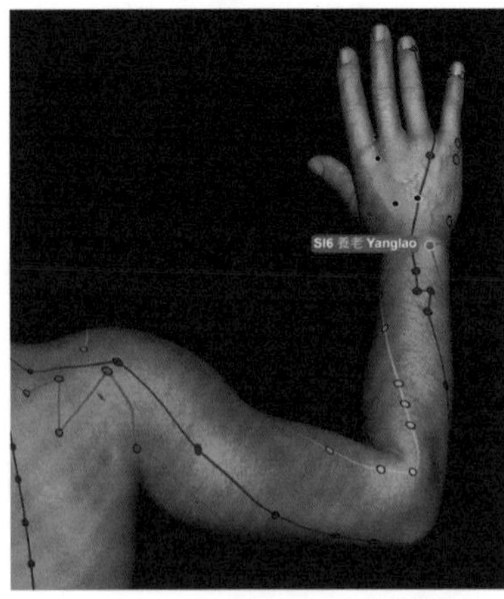

SI 6: YANG LAO (NURSING THE AGED)

Name: Nursing the Aged, Helps deal with aging when our yang decreases.

Location: When the palm faces the chest, the points is in the hollow on the radial side of the styloid process of the ulna

Indication:

1. It is an important point for the growth of yang qi, enjoying old age - life.
2. Improve eyesight.
3. Relax neck and shoulder muscles.

It is mainly used for hand numbness, dizziness, and shoulder pain. It is commonly used in modern times to treat vision loss, eye hyperemia, hemiplegia, acute lumbar sprain, stiff neck, etc. If you want to keep your eyes healthy, you need to massage these two points regularly.

Techniques and notes: Massage this acupoint with fingers or Jade board Guasha board. to improve eyesight and soothe the nerves.

Miscellaneous bits:

Element: Fire
Direction: South
Season: Summer
Climate: Heat

Sense Organ: Tongue
Sense: Touch
Number of Acupoints: 19 on one side of the body, total 38.

Small Intestine Meditation

When you are comfortable, I would like you to gently close your eyes and focus your attention onto the sound of my voice.

As you listen now, I would like you to become aware of your body and how your clothes feel against your skin.

Can you imagine feeling completely relaxed? I wonder if you could take a nice deep breath in, and as you release the breath slowly, let go of all the tension in those muscles around your body.

You already know how to breathe deeply so allow yourself to enjoy all the sensations of a deep breath in and breathing out all the tensions as you relax.

Short pause.

As your breathing returns to its normal pace, you know that each gentle out-breath can lead to more and more relaxation.

Paying attention to your breathing can help you relax even more.

This is your own special time that you have set aside just for you, because you don't need to be anywhere or do anything apart from concentrate on your breathing and relax all those muscles.

Any sounds you may hear around you only serve to take you deeper and deeper, knowing that you can return to your normal state of consciousness if you need to.

There is no time, but now, there is no place but here and right now and right here, you are safe, supported and relaxed. Sooner or later, you'll find yourself wondering about going into an even deeper state of relaxation, and you may do that suddenly or gradually.

As you do this, you feel your body becoming heavier and heavier as every muscle in your body begins to let go as you sink deeper – and deeper

– into this wonderful feeling of peace and tranquility...

Your body is so comfortable and knows that it is safe and supported...

And I wonder if you will allow yourself to truly - let go - as you go deeper and deeper into relaxation...

As you do, allow your mind to drift away, now; you are slowing down, feeling more at ease and even more relaxed.

Pause.

Take another slow deep breath, hold it to the count of three… release and relax...

Imagine now if you will, that you are walking down a trail. You come upon a river. The river of your life.

At the river bank there is a canoe.

Climb into the canoe and paddle out into the middle of the stream. Pull the paddle in and allow yourself to float and drift along.

Feel a gentle breeze in your face ... Feel the warm sun...

Sit back and look up into the beautiful blue sky, just the shade of blue you like so much.

Notice white puffy clouds drifting across the sky, sometimes taking shapes you recognize, sometimes not.

Smell the river smell.

Smell the muddy banks and the pine trees in the distance.

See the trees, shrubs and flowers along the bank.

Notice the bees and butterflies… they somehow know just how to get at the sweet nectar inside.

Drift ... Float...

Harmonize the rhythm of your body with the river of your life and the earth mother… vibrate as one, in sync with nature and your human nature at once and touch base with your higher self as you prepare for a journey of transformation… into the world of joy and happiness…

Meet your higher self and prepare for a meditative journey…

Let us turn the meditation now toward observing your breathing, and slowly become aware of the impermanence of your breathing.

Each breath is different from the one that came before it, and is different from the one that comes after it... You are breathing in different air with each breath, and your body is changing with each breath... there are different sensations around the nose and inside the nostrils... your lungs expand and contract, your abdomen rises and falls... Each breath is just a breath, neither a good breath nor a bad breath...

So, in each moment, with each breath, there is change, flux and flow... Then think about other changes that are taking place in your body in each moment... Think of how your body is made of many different parts—arms, legs, head, skin, blood, bones, nerves and muscles, organs and meridians like the small intestine meridian... and how these parts themselves are made of yet smaller parts, such as cells... Become aware of the movement that is going on each moment... the beating of your heart, the flow of your blood, the circulation of your qi and the energy of your nerve-impulses... On a more subtle level, cells are being born, moving about, dying and disintegrating...

On an even subtler level... all the parts of your body are made of molecules, atoms and sub-atomic particles, and these are in constant motion... Try to really get a feeling for the change that is taking place each moment in your body.... This will help you begin to understand qi...

Feel how your awareness of your meridians empowers you to alter your body's balance; how your meridian awareness can provide the opportunity to not only shift from wherever you are to balance and harmony, but also to project love and kindness to others...

Visualize the small intestine meridian starting from the tip of the little finger and crosses the palm and wrist... It runs upwards along the posterior side of the forearm until it reaches the back of the shoulder where it ends at the uppermost part of the back at the bottom of the neck...

At this position, it first branches off and moves internally through the heart and stomach to reach the small intestine... The second branch travels externally across the neck and cheek until it reaches the outer corner of the eye and then enters the ear... A short branch in the cheek moves upward to the inner corner of the eye where it connects with the bladder meridian.

At the bottom of the neck the meridian enters an area known as the "Empty Basin," the top of shoulder area.... It first branches off and moves internally through the heart and stomach to reach the small intestine…

Embrace the opportunity to nurture your small intestine meridian… know that the small intestine is responsible for receiving food during the digestion process, the small intestine is known as the Minister of Reception… It separates impurities from the food before passing the waste on and also absorbs water ...

One of the functions of the small intestine is the body's main absorption, kind of like the IRS, collecting the money and absorbing the essence ... It collects a lot of good things, but it can't use it by itself ... It must take out its essence and turn it over to the "treasury", and then Yuanqi, prenatal qi will be the administrator and expenditure officer of the treasury...

Then turn your attention to your psyche ... It too is composed of many parts… thoughts, perceptions, feelings, memories, images… following one after the other, ceaselessly… Spend a few minutes simply observing the ever-changing flow of experiences in your mind, like surfing through many different web pages…

Don't cling to anything that you see in your mind, don't judge or make comments… just observe, and try to get a sense of the neutral, ever-changing nature of your mind…

After reflecting on the neutrality of your inner world… your own body and mind… extend your awareness to the outer world… Think about your immediate surroundings… the cushion, mat or bed you are sitting on… the floor, walls, windows and ceiling of the room you are sitting in… the furniture and other objects in the room… Consider that each of these things, although appearing different from each other, is actually a neutral thing, one not having greater value than the other…

Stay with that awareness of the neutral, constantly-changing nature of these things ... Then let your awareness travel further out… beyond the walls of your room… Think of other people… their bodies and minds are also neutral, none inherently better than another… The same is true of all living beings, such as animals, birds and insects ...

Think of all the inanimate objects in the world and in the universe: houses, buildings, roads, cars, trees, mountains, oceans and rivers, the earth itself, the sun, moon and stars ... All of these things, being composed of atoms and other minute particles, are constantly changing, every moment, every millisecond and each have their own value ... Nothing is better than something else except for the value that our ego gives it ... While you are meditating, if at any point you experience a clear, strong feeling of the neutral nature of things, stop the thinking or analyzing process, and hold your attention firmly on this feeling ... Concentrate on it for as long as possible… without thinking of anything else or letting your mind be distracted ...

When the feeling fades or your attention starts to wander, again return to analyzing the neutral nature of things...

Concentrate on the thought that it is unrealistic and self-defeating to cling to things with our ego ... Whatever is beautiful and pleasing has been assigned that value by our ego… so we can't expect it to give us lasting happiness ... Also, whatever is unpleasant or disturbing has also been assigned that value by our ego… it might even change if we change our perspective!… So there's no need to judge or to reject it...

Dedicate the positive energy from doing this meditation that you and all others in this group will find perfect happiness and freedom from understanding that we have egos and shadows and in getting to know those aspects of ourselves move into a psychological rebirth as we reach integration and individuation...

Fully understand that with practice, meditation itself can become the venue for manifesting and the discovery and development of you ... learning to observe yourself and your thoughts can be the first step toward moving away from powerless states of mind and a belief that external forces control you toward an empowered state of knowing yourself…

Give yourself permission to embrace a new awareness of your power to create reality through the balancing of your meridians, through meditation and how this awareness will prepare you to live unconditionally…

Draw your attention to the warmth in your heart now… like a ripple in a pond, a ripple of inner awareness, notice how it feels to be encased in that ripple… feel a sense of your increased knowing transmuting into warmth to a dozen others…

Bring your awareness to the smile on your face as you realize that the meaning of life just may be to become who you came here to be and that becoming permeates your body, mind and soul…

Now that you are coming through all of this, notice the happiness you feel inside knowing how powerful meridian balance is and how connected to humanity you are…notice how this connection fills you with an elevated vibration… and how an elevated vibration can expand the visible spectrums of your senses…

Now just breathe and be with yourself and let the waves of your breathing be with you…

CHAPTER SEVEN

Bladder Meridian

Characteristics

The bladder is referred to as the "Minister of the Reservoir," the official of the management of the reservoir that collects, stores, transfers and distributes the body's fluids to the rest of the body. It is also known as the Tai Yang Meridian.

The bladder works in conjunction with the kidney to extract nutritional essence from bodily fluids. After extraction, transformation and distribution of the Qi, the bladder stores urine for elimination.

The longest meridian in front of the human body is the stomach meridian, the longest meridian of the back is the bladder meridian, and the longest one of the two sides is the gallbladder meridian. So these three meridians are all substantial elements of the energetic aspect of the human body.

From three pm to five pm, meridian Qi mainly flows through the Bladder meridian. This is the best time to work and study.

Time for efficient work and a good time to drink tea.

Drink lots of water, too. Detox!

The Minister of the Reservoir collects, stores, transfers and distributes bodily fluids to the rest of the body.

In TCM, the bladder is so much more than the Western medicine concept of urine storage. And, urine doesn't just flow out, it should be sprayed out. The healthy bladder with plenty of Yang Qi sprays urine. When you are young and Yang Qi is sufficient and bladder Qi is fully transformed, urine will spray far. When you get old, your Yang Qi declines, and your urine tends to drip.

The kidney and the bladder are very closely related. The kidney controls storage, but the bladder performs the function of storage. Body fluids contain the nutrition of the human body, the Jing. But these nutrients must be extracted.

The kidneys store the essence, but the bladder meridian transforms the essence, refining the Jing and transforming the body fluids to Jing and Qi. Transformation and distribution are the most important functions of the bladder meridian.

While the organ stores and eliminates liquid waste, excreting urine with help from kidney Qi, the energetic function involves balancing the autonomic nervous system. The bladder meridian connects and awakens the Jing (essence) in the brain. This is in part because the bladder meridian spans the height of the body and runs alongside the spinal column. The bladder plays a role in regulating the sympathetic and parasympathetic responses.

Bladder Meridian

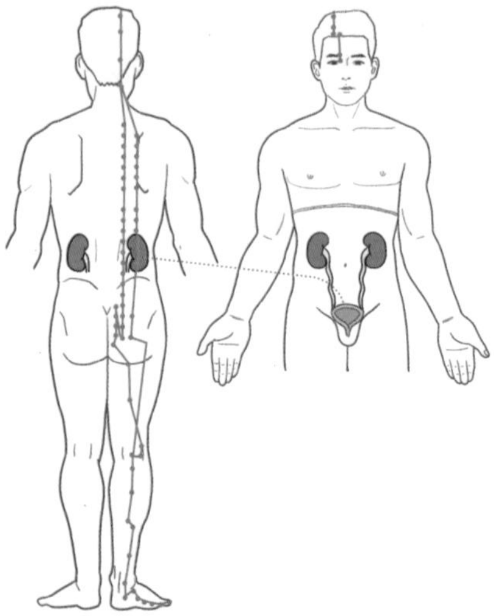

Primary Pathway

The small intestine ends at the inner side of the eye. The bladder begins in the inner side of the eye, both are connected in the inner side of the eye.

The bladder meridian starts at the inner side of the eye and goes across the forehead to reach the top of the head where it branches into the brain. The main channel then goes across the back of the head and divides into two branches. One branch crosses the center of the base of the neck and extends downwards parallel to the spine.

Once in the lumbar region (bottom of the spine), it branches out to reach the bladder. The other branch crosses the back of the shoulder and runs downward on the outside, which is adjacent and parallel to the inner branch. It continues down until it reaches the buttocks where two branches run across the back of the thigh along different pathways that join at the back of the knee.

The joint meridian then continues along the back of the lower leg, circles behind the outer ankle, runs along the outside of the foot and terminates on the lateral side of the tip of the small toe, where it connects with the kidney meridian.

The main channel goes across the acupuncture points in this meridian, which are indicated for diseases in the head, neck, eyes, back, groin and lower limbs as well as certain mental illnesses. They are also recommended for symptoms along the meridian pathway.

An imbalance of the bladder meridian can cause lower back pain or lower back weakness as well as urinary problems. A bladder meridian imbalance can also cause one to be fearful or stubborn.

The acupoints of this meridian can mainly treat diseases of the urogenital system, mental, nervous system, respiratory system, circulatory system, digestive system and diseases of the parts where this meridian passes. For example: epilepsy, headache, eye disease, nasal disease, enuresis, dysuria and pain in the back of the lower limbs, etc.

The bladder meridian of foot Taiyang is the longest of the fourteen meridians. It is also the meridian with the most acupoints. There are 67 acupoints on each side of this meridian, with 134 acupoints total on the left and right. Among them, 49 acupoints are distributed on the head, face, neck and back, and 18 acupoints are distributed on the midline behind the lower limbs and the outer part of the feet. The first point is the Jingming point, and the last point is the Zhi yin point.

A blood transfusion can illustrate the concept of transformation. Why can't a blood transfusion be directly injected instead of drop by drop? Life is at risk if the drip is too fast. The blood must be transformed by your body to become your own. Drops of liquid medicine and blood are foreign objects to our bodies. We can't transform them if they drop too quickly. Life needs to transform, to merge, and to assimilate.

Imbalanced, difficult transformation requires us to spend our perinatal Qi. When we are sick our perinatal Qi is already weak. If the installation speed is too fast, the person will not be able to bear it, and the whole body will become progressively colder, and even die.

Yang transformation is essential to life.

Essence and Spirit are also transformed into each other.

The theory of five elements explains how Qi cycles through various stages of transformation. As Yin and Yang continuously adjust to one another and transform into one another in a never-ending dance of harmonization, they tend to do so in a predictable pattern.

Each phase of transformation gives birth to, and nourishes, the next phase in sequence.

Each phase of transformation also has a restraining influence on the phase opposite to it. By increasing or decreasing the qualities and functions associated with a particular phase, a practitioner may either nourish a phase that is in deficiency or drain a phase that is in excess or restrain a phase that is exerting too much influence.

When the organs have sufficient Yang Qi normal metabolism follows, which promotes Qi transformation. For example, if the small intestine is full of Qi, the human body can absorb nutrients well; if the bladder is full of Qi, people are less likely to get sick.

Exercise can promote transformation of the human body. Today, many people experience problems related to sedentary lifestyles.

Passion, lust, physical labor, etc., can also promote the transformations of "essence." If people feel that life is boring and their mood is low, their ability to facilitate transformation is stagnated and weak.

Main Indication

Disharmony of the bladder meridian can lead to dysfunction. This dysfunction is often related to symptoms caused by external pernicious influences that can cause disease such as cold, wind, fire, dampness, dryness and summer heat.

Symptoms

Because the Tai Yang meridian is considered the most exterior, it is the first meridian to be invaded if there is any external attack. Therefore, its disharmony can cause symptoms such as difficult urination, incontinence, painful eyes, runny nose, nose bleeding and nasal congestion.

Headache, neck, back, groin and buttock areas indicate disharmony in the bladder meridian pathway.

Migraines and rushing headaches, like a swollen blood vessel rushing upward (which are also related to liver blood deficiency). The blood vessels are elastic and belong to the tendons. The bladder is responsible for the tendon problems, and the reason is that the tendons cannot be nourished by the blood. Furthermore, the bladder is the Yang, and if the Yang is empty, the Qi will rush upwards, causing emptiness headaches. Some people often have a headache before menstruation. The brow is exactly the Jing point of the bladder meridian. The lower Jiao blood is congested and the upper Jiao blood is insufficient. This can also be the case.

Headache with eye pressure: The eyes seem to fall off and pull out. This headache can cause bulging eyes and a stiff neck. This disease is also like hyperthyroidism, which is rooted in the liver and kidney, and is also related to Yang deficiency of the bladder meridian. In this case, you can massage the bladder meridian and the shoulders, and the neck will feel better. If the neck is cold all the time, it can also be more comfortable to apply a hot towel or blow it with a hair dryer. Jade Guasha board can also be used for scraping on the neck and other parts. The most important thing is daily maintenance.

Back pain is a symptom of bladder meridian dysfunction. This shows up when your back and hips cannot bend. The bladder meridian travels through the back and waist. When the bladder is cold, it will cause back pain. The waist seems to be broken.

At the same time, the hip bones are not flexible. The pain is deep. One way to avoid these problems is to keep yourself warm. Another is to have someone massage your legs and back every day and open the bladder meridian.

Other symptoms include: madness, epilepsy, mental problems and hemorrhoids.

The bladder governs problems with the tendons. The tendon energy shows up in our nails and fingers, that is, the problem of tendons can also be known from the external nails and fingers and toes.

Each meridian has associated tendons and associated diseases. So body fluid cannot be transformed or transmitted, and people will have contractions of the tendons and veins.

After getting older, leg cramps often occur in the middle of the night, which is related to insufficient transformation of the bladder.

Understand the bladder meridian transformational processes.

Understanding the transformational process of the bladder meridian will help you understand much more. When transformations are weak, there is less urine output, because the generation of urine also depends on bladder transformation. Insufficient Yang Qi translates into an inability to hold back your need to urinate and/or frequent urination. Thinking too much will deplete the Yang Qi. You can see that young people think less about things, have enough Qi and blood, and have enough Yang Qi, and they can pee up to the wind. When people get old, their Yang Qi is insufficient and their power of recuperation is also weak. Many people suffer from urinary incontinence. When an older person coughs sometimes urine can be expelled.

Why do women have more "urinary incontinence" than men? The first thing to consider is the difference between men and women. Men are Yang, women are Yin, and the ability to absorb is a function of Yang. Women are inherently weaker in this regard. Second, the reason why women have to squat to pee is because women basically rely on lung breathing. The man breathes from his belly, so standing up to urinate can exert his strength. When people get old, lung Qi will be deficient before kidney Qi, so women have more urinary incontinence than men. But men suffer more from prostate problems.

The biggest problem of weak transformations is that it is easy to cause dampness and puffiness. Chinese· medicine does not think obesity is a disease, but that dampness is a disease, and what can really change dampness must be the power of true Yang Qi. On the other hand, the overweight man without dampness has a ruddy complexion, a soft temperament, and is still as light as a swallow.

The water in the human body is divided into three states in the triple warmer of the human body. The upper burner (upper body) is like a fog, that is, the water in the upper body/warmer is in a state of fog/cloud/light moistness, which generally does not condense. If the water is condensed, it will also cause swelling of the upper eyelid and bags under the eyes. The water in the middle body/ warmer is a swamp state. If the spleen is not transported and transformed properly, it will become a dampness evil. Generally, TCM will use Atractylodes (Bai Zhu) and other herbal medicines to specifically drum up the waist and navel to relieve dampness. The lower warmer of the human body is a state of rushing like a river. Here, the Yang Qi transformations of the small intestine and bladder are especially needed to prevent dampness from being formed.

So what can promote the transformations of the human body?

1) The true Yang of the kidney can transform "essence" into Qi; the essence of the kidney can transform into Qi, that is, true fire generates true earth, "essence" supplies the spleen and stomach, and the spleen controls the muscles. On the other hand, if a person has no energy, either the essence is insufficient, or the kidney essence cannot be transformed into Qi. Furthermore, the kidney essence is mainly responsible for storage, but if there is a problem with the function of the kidney, it may contain garbage, and if the bladder meridian is insufficient and the Qi is incapable of transforming, it may form kidney stones.

2) The organs have sufficient Yang Qi and normal metabolism, which can promote Qi transformation. For example, if the small intestine is full of Qi, the human body can absorb nutrients well; if the bladder is full of Qi, people are less likely to get sick.
3) Exercise can promote the transformation of the human body. Many people's problems nowadays are related to sedentary and excessive staying at home.
4) Passion, lust, physical labor, etc. can also promote the transformations of "essence." If people feel that life is boring and their mood is low, their ability to facilitate transformations is stagnant and weak. In fact, travel, fishing, and love are life, work is life. Unfortunately, most people's lives are just repetitive work.

Acupoints

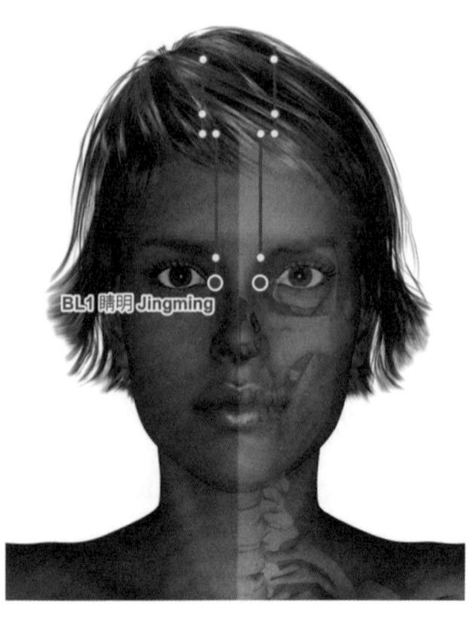

UB 1 JING MING (EYE'S CLARITY)

Name: Eye's Clarity, also called "Bright Eyes," this point improves eyesight. A very powerful point, it will improve both inner and outer sight as it is an intersection of many pathways. When Yin and Yang are in harmony we have clarity and brightness. Sun and moon gives understanding. Putting light into the Jing (the mystery).

Location: 0.1 cun superior to the inner canthus of the eye.

Indication: Redness, swelling, pain in eyes, itching of eyes, night blindness, color blindness, blurry vision, dim vision, nearsightedness, hormonal issues, low energy, dizziness.

Because Jingming acupoint belongs to the bladder meridian, it can also treat acute low back pain and tachycardia.

Techniques and notes: Massage with fingers. Moxibustion is prohibited at this point.

*It is the hand-Taiyang small intestine, foot-Taiyang bladder, foot-Yangming stomach, Yinqiao, Yangqiao five meridian meeting points.

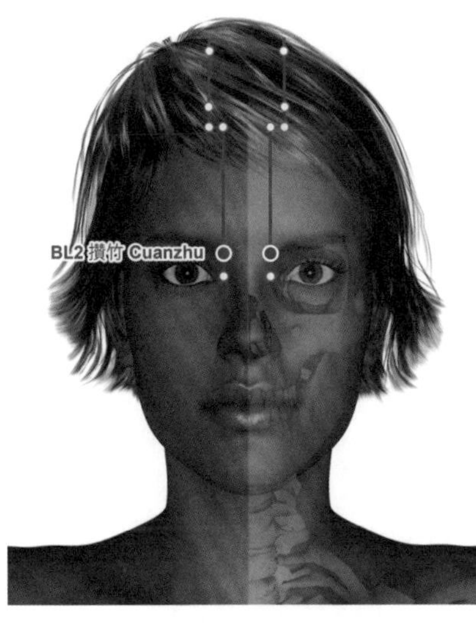

UB 2: ZAN ZHU (COLLECTING BAMBOO)

Name: Collecting bamboo: Gathered bamboo looks like an eyebrow.

Location: On the medial extremity of the eyebrow, or in the supraorbital notch.

Indication: Headache, blurring and failing vision, pain in supraorbital region, lacrimation, redness, pain in eyes, eyelid twitching, glaucoma, tearing in the wind, facial paralysis, etc.

Frowning eyebrows: Frowning is to adjust Yang Qi to help you think about things, so eyebrows are the expression of Yang Qi. The inner eyebrows are Tai Yang bladder meridian, the middle of the eyebrows is the Yangming stomach meridian, and outer of the eyebrows are the Shaoyang Sanjiao and the small intestine meridian, Therefore, if the eyebrows are high and thick, it means the yang qi is open and expend, and if the eyebrows are low and thin, the yang qi is reserved.

If a person has skin blemishes in the eyebrow area it likely means that the starting point of the bladder meridian is blocked and there is likely a problem with the bladder meridian.

A frown can be a visible sign that we are encountering problems in life, our eye brows narrow when thinking about a problem. A result of this activity is to mobilize yang qi. When you press and rub the brow bone carefully, you will find two small pits. These pits are the starting points of the bladder meridian. Regular massage of these two points will make your eyes bright and activate yang qi. If the yang qi is insufficient, it will go up along the middle line of the bridge of the nose, forming vertical lines between the brows, which is also a sign of a lack of yang qi.

The key to a harmonious mind is to be able to think clearly and to be transparent with your heart, which guards against stress between the brain and heart.

It is important to understand that you can make yourself sick by fretting about problems. Breathe deeply and align your brain and heart to work through issues.

Headache: Pain at the top of the head is due to deficiency of liver blood and yang-qi in the bladder; headache in the eyebrows is due to deficiency of Yang-qi in the bladder meridian; the entire forehead pain is due to the stomach meridian problem; headache like a circle band around the head is due to dampness in the spleen, which is also related to Dai Mai meridian.

Neck Pain: The bladder meridian runs from the brain to the back of the neck and the upper shoulder. Therefore, the first likely cause of neck pain is Yang deficiency because the cervical vertebra goes through the governor vessel and the Bladder Meridian, and with insufficient Yang Qi the cervical vertebra becomes dystrophic.

The second is long-term improper posture and overwork. For example, bowing the head for a long time will make the neck muscles tense and strained. People are always looking down at the mobile phone, which is a problem. Over time, the neck will have a big bump and become a "turtleneck." A large bag will bulge in the neck blocking the meridians causing headache and memory loss. Lying in bed at night and checking the phone will cause neck stiffness, numbness in the arms, and the eyes get tired.

The third is to suffer from a cold. The cervical vertebra is in the yang position, and is negatively affected by cold, so pay attention to keeping warm. Always a good idea in winter to wear a scarf.

Techniques and notes: Massage with fingers

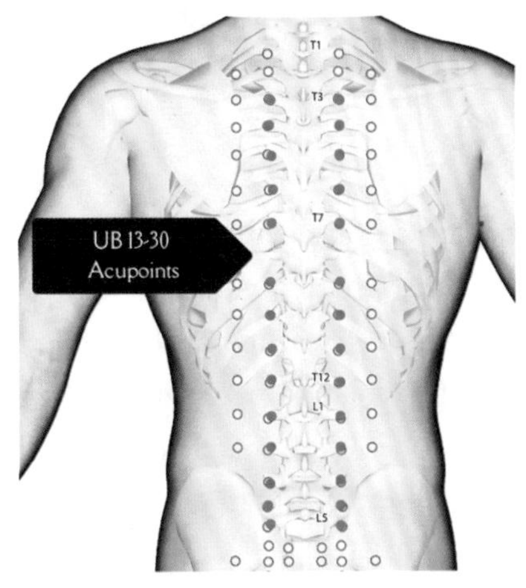

UB 13 - 30: UB BACK ACUPOINTS

Location: From the first thoracic vertebra to the two sides below the spinous process of the fifth lumbar vertebra, 1.5 cun lateral to the posterior midline.

There are 17 acupoints on one side, and a total of 34 acupoints on the left and right, including Lung's Shu, Absolute Yin Shu, Heart's Shu, Governing Shu, Diaphragm's Shu, Liver's Shu, Gall Bladder's Shu, Spleen's Shu, Stomach Shu, Triple Burner's Shu, Kidney's Shu, etc.

Indication: These are very important points that are commonly used to treat diseases of the corresponding internal organs, such as vascular headache, acroparesthesia, autonomic dysfunction syndrome, cerebrovascular disease, erythematous extremity pain, hypertension, etc. In ancient times, there was a saying that, "Once Jia Ji has been unblocked, there won't be any illness in the body." The bladder meridian is the core of human meridians, and the Du meridian is the commander of the Yang meridian. Jiaji acupoint passes through the Du meridian and communicates with the bladder meridian.

Among them, Kidney's Shu UB 23 can treat enuresis, dysuria, edema; nocturnal emission, impotence, irregular menstruation, leucorrhea; deafness, tinnitus, cough, asthma; stroke, hemiplegia, low back pain, bone disease, etc.

Large Intestine Shu UB 25 can treat bloating, diarrhea, constipation, bleeding hemorrhoids; low back pain; urticarial, etc.

Small Intestine Shu UB 27 can treat lumbosacral pain, knee pain, abdominal pain, dysuria, nocturnal emission, leucorrhea, etc.

Techniques and notes: To stimulate Jiaji acupoints, you can press and knead them. Use the thumbs of both hands to push and knead the Jiaji acupoints from top to bottom along both sides of the spine for 5 minutes. The pain points should be rubbed more. Long-term massage of the

Jiaji acupoints can prevent many internal organ diseases. Moxibustion and Jade Guasha scraping can also be used.

UB 31- 34: EIGHT LIAO POINTS:

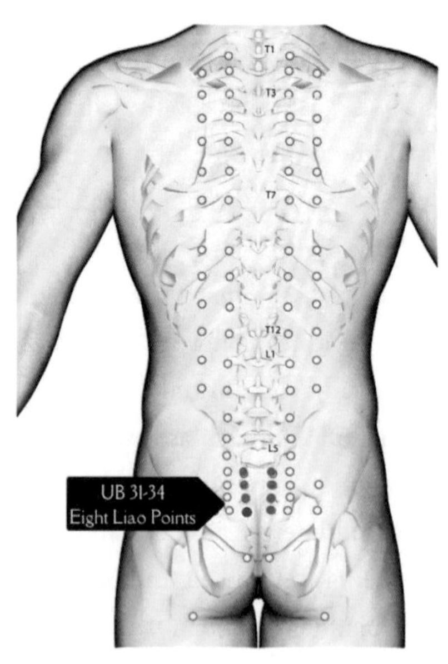

Location: located in the first, second, third and fourth posterior sacral foramen. There are eight acupoints on the left and right, namely Upper Bone Hole BU 31, Second Bone Hole UB 32, Middle Bone Hole UB 33, Lower Bone Hole UB 34.

Indications: lumbosacral diseases, low back pain, sciatica, lower limb paralysis, dysuria, irregular menstruation, lower abdominal pain, constipation, pelvic inflammatory disease and other diseases.

This area is adjacent to the uterus. The flesh in this area should be very soft and can be pinched. If it is not soft, it means that there is adhesion between the meridians and the skin. This adhesion is the external manifestation of a problem in the body, especially the uterus, and all gynecological diseases are closely connected with the uterus.

Acupuncture, Tuina, massage, cupping or moxibustion in the eight-liao area is to regulate the uterus from the outside to the inside. The eight Liao is where the nerves and blood vessels that govern the internal organs of the pelvis converge. The uterus is healthy, gynecological problems are gone, and many miscellaneous diseases that plague women, such as insomnia, constipation, anger, impatience, laziness, etc., will disappear naturally.

Techniques and notes: Acupuncture, Tuina, massage, cupping or moxibustion.

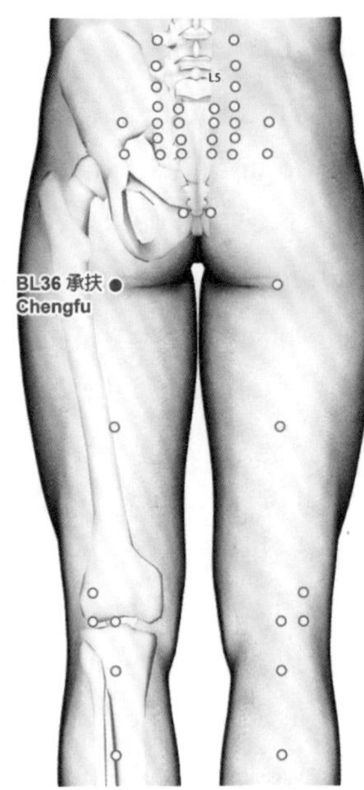

UB 36: CHENG FU (BEARING SUPPORT)

Name: Bearing Support, to transfer and disperse the stress of a situation, to put things in order.

Location: On the posterior aspect of the thigh, in the middle of the transverse gluteal fold. It is located on the back of the thigh, at the midpoint of the horizontal crease below the buttocks.

Indications: Low back, hip and femoral pain, hemorrhoids, constipation and so on.

If the buttocks are cold, you can also massage the Chengfu point, push the Chengfu point upward, and can also lift the buttocks.

Techniques and notes: Massage

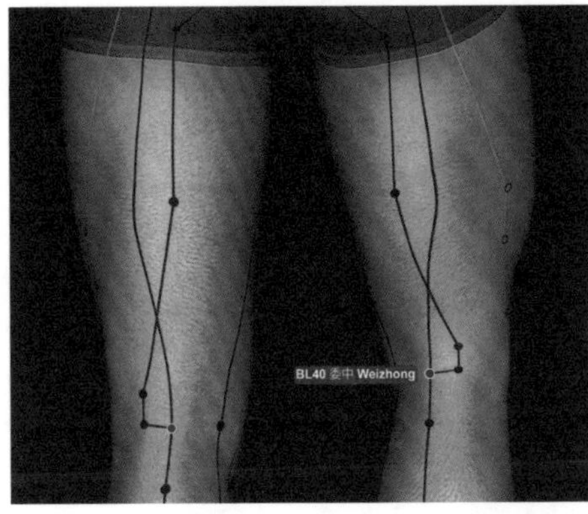

UB 40: WEI ZHONG (BEND MIDDLE)

Name: Bend Middle, middle of the back of knee. Earth point.

Location: Midpoint of transverse crease of the popliteal fossa, between the tendon of m. biceps femoris and m. semitendinosus.

Indication: lower back can use acupuncture or massage Weizhong point. It also treats headaches because the bladder meridian enters the brain. It is easy to have nodes in the tendon in the popliteal fossa, and tendon knots hinder the essence and qi. When a person gets old, his legs get old first. It can also treat hemiplegia, paralysis of the lower limbs, erysipelas, and itching all over the body.

Techniques and notes: Massage

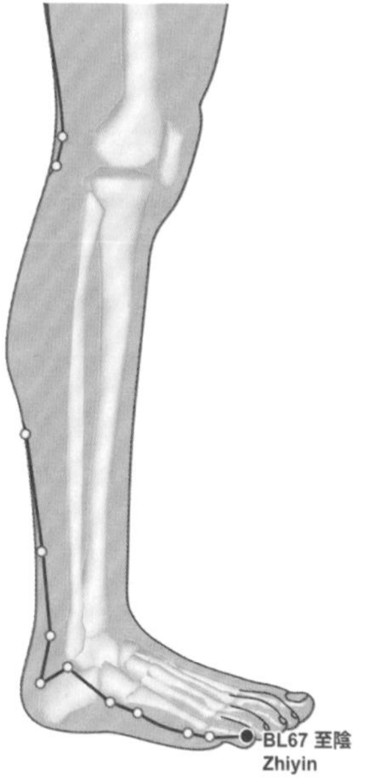

UB 67 ZHI YIN (REACHING YIN)

Name: Reaching Yin, when yin reaches its extreme. Last point on the channel, when the bladder becomes the kidney channel and ends at the Gate of Life.
Location: 0.1 cun posterior to the corner of the nail, on the lateral aspect of the small toe.
Indication: Headache, dizziness. TCM says that the upper disease is treated by lower body acupoints. The root of the bladder meridian lies in the yin and is connected with the kidney meridian. Insufficient kidney essence can cause headache or dizziness. Acupuncture to the yin point can relieve the symptoms.

Malposition of the fetus and difficult labor. For example, if the fetus is in a transverse or breech position in the mother's womb, or an overdue baby. In ancient China, there were midwives who would massage the abdomen and moxibustion the Zhi yin point, to help deliver the baby naturally. Now, in the western countries, the C- section is a common solution. I have helped so many breech and overdue moms, by using Zhi Yin points to have natural delivery and avoid C-section. Sometimes I will teach family members to moxa this point.
Itching in the genitals: There are two periods of itching in the genitals of young women. One is the ovulation period, which belongs to the growth of yang qi; another time is the beginning and end of the period, this is because of blood deficiency. Danggui Sini Decoction combined with acupuncture or moxibustion Zhi Yin point is very useful.

Nasal obstruction, malposition feverish sensation in sole.

Blurred vision, pain in eye.

Stiff neck.

Miscellaneous bits

Element: Water
Direction: North
Season: Winter
Climate: Cold
Sense Organ: Ears
Sense: Hearing
Tissue: Bones
Positive Emotion: Gentleness
Negative Emotion: Fear
Opposite: Lung
Yin/Yang: Yang
Flow Direction: Down
Origin/Ending: Face to Foot
Number of Acupoints: 67 on one side, 134 total.

Bladder Meditation

When you are comfortable, I would like you to gently close your eyes and focus your attention onto the sound of my voice.

As you listen now, I would like you to become aware of your body and how your clothes feel against your skin.

Can you imagine feeling completely relaxed? I wonder if you could take a nice deep breath in, and as you release the breath slowly, let go of all the tension in those muscles around your body.

Give yourself permission to enjoy all the sensations of a deep breath in and then, exhale out all the tensions as you relax.

Short pause.

Let's go on a sacred meditative journey of transformation…

As totally relaxed as you are - you are also aware that you can hear my voice clearly - more clearly than before.

And should you hear any other noises - outside sounds in the busy world left far behind - they will merge into the background - they will not disturb you.

So, right now - as you have your eyes closed - I want you to allow yourself to pretend that you cannot open them - that's right - pretend that you cannot open your eyes - and keep on pretending.

And while you are pretending you cannot open your eyes - you will try momentarily to open your eyes and you will find that it is impossible.

Of course, it is you concentrating hard on your pretense that prevents you from opening your eyes - because you know very well that you could open your eyes anytime that you choose to stop pretending.

Now when you are sure that your eyes are so relaxed - that as long as you hang onto this relaxation they just won't work - then hold onto that relaxation.

Now this relaxation that you have in your eyes is the same level of relaxation that you have throughout your entire body.

Feel that level and quality of relaxation spreading throughout your entire body.

And as you relish in your peaceful feeling, let your mind drift to the magic of the meridians and how they work like a network system, transporting and distributing Qi and blood ... how the meridians link up organs, limbs, joints, bones, tendons, tissues and skin, and provide communication between the body interior and exterior, through a healthy meridian system...

Marvel at the magic of how Qi and blood successfully warm and nourish different organs and tissues, and maintain normal metabolic activities...

Understand that meridians are essential in supporting the flow of nutritive Qi inside the blood vessels and flow of protective Qi around them ... they strengthen the body's immunity, protect against external pernicious influences and assist in regulating Yin and Yang ...

Know that the bladder is referred to as the Minister of the Reservoir, the official of the management of the reservoir that collects, stores, transfers and distributes the body's fluids to the rest of the body...

Returning now to your breath, you know that each gentle out-breath can lead to more and more relaxation...

Paying attention to your breathing can help you relax even more...

Know that the bladder works in conjunction with the kidney to extract nutritional essence from bodily fluids. After extraction, transformation and distribution of the qi, the bladder stores urine for elimination...

Understand that from 3 pm to 5 pm, meridian Qi mainly flows through the Bladder meridian, this is the best time to work and study ... this is time for efficient work and a good time to drink tea ... you should also drink lots of water, too ... Detox!

Right now is your own special time that you have set aside just for you, because you don't need to be anywhere or do anything apart from concentrate on your breathing and relax all those muscles ...

There is no time, but now, there is no place but here and right now and right here, you are safe, supported and relaxed ... sooner or later, you'll find yourself wondering about going into an even deeper state of relaxation, and you may do that suddenly or gradually...

As you do this, you feel your body becoming heavier and heavier as every muscle in your body begins to let go as you sink deeper – and deeper – into this wonderful feeling of peace and tranquility...

Allow that in Traditional Chinese Medicine the bladder is so much more than the Western medicine concept of urine storage ... while the kidneys store the essence, the bladder meridian transforms the essence, refining the Jing and transforming the body fluids to Jing and Qi ... transformation and distribution are the most important functions of the bladder meridian ...

Visualize balanced transformation throughout your body, your meridians and especially your bladder meridian…

Know that as yin and yang continuously adjust to one another and transform into one another there is a never-ending dance of harmonization… when the organs have sufficient yang qi normal metabolism follows, which promotes qi transformation ... if the bladder is full of qi, you are less likely to get sick ...

Set your intention to grow awareness of your power of meridian balance and harmony and understand that you can resist being carried along on a current not of your own making… resist blaming external forces for anything in your life… instead shaping your experience by setting your intention to achieve what you want and by extension affect your outer world experience…

Accept that the key to a harmonious mind is to be able to think clearly and to be transparent with your heart… which guards against stress between the brain and heart ... understanding that you can make yourself sick by fretting about problems ....

Breathe deeply and align your brain and heart to work through issues ... Prepare for making the unconscious conscious through meditation, which will result in balanced meridians, enhanced focus, increased emotional intelligence, greater mental strength, improved physical health, healthy relationships and ultimately to self-realization…

Give yourself permission to embrace a new awareness of your power to create reality through the balancing of your meridians, through meditation and how this awareness will prepare you to live unconditionally…

notice the happiness you feel inside knowing how powerful meridian balance is and how connected to humanity you are…notice how this connection fills you with an elevated vibration… and how an elevated vibration can expand the visible spectrums of your senses…

Now just breathe and be with yourself and let the waves of your breathing be with you…

CHAPTER EIGHT

Kidney Meridian

Characteristics

The kidney is known as the "Minister of Power." It is tasked with storing the prenatal energy as well as the essential vital energy for life.

Also known as the "mansion of fire and water," and the "residence of Yin and Yang," the kidney also works at regulating the brain and plays an important role in the formation of memories and rationality.

From five pm to seven pm, meridian Qi mainly flows through the kidney meridian, this is the best time to eat your dinner and restore your energy.

Kidneys store energy reserves.

Be sure to put yourself first when it comes to your energy.

In TCM, the kidney is seen as one of the most important organs. This organ includes the adrenal glands and the male and female sex.

As noted, it is known as the "Minister of Power" from whom ingenuity is derived, an official who protects the monarch's "heart," as well as the "Root of Life."

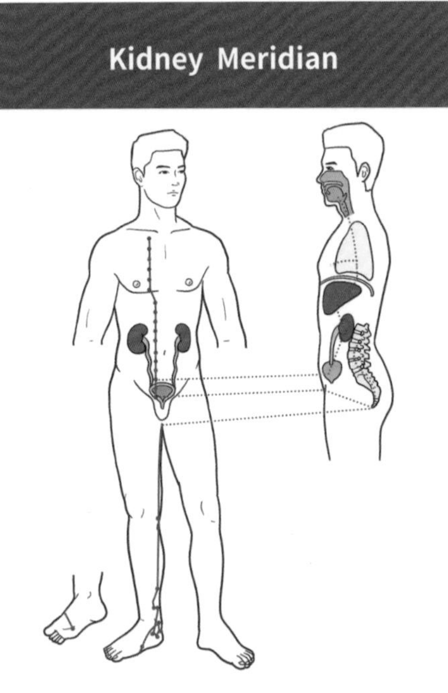

Primary Pathway

The Kidney Meridian starts from the inferior side of the small toe. Crossing the middle of the sole and the arch of the foot, it circles behind the inner ankle and travels along the innermost side of the lower leg and thigh, until it enters the body near the base of the backbone.

After connecting with the kidney, it comes out at the pubic bone. Over the abdomen, it runs externally upwards until it reaches the upper part of the chest (the inner side of the clavicle).

A second branch emerges from the kidney and moves internally upwards and passes through the liver, diaphragm, lungs and throat, finally terminating at the root of the tongue. Another small branch divides from the lung to connect with the heart and the pericardium.

The functions of the kidneys:

The kidney's main function is to protect the monarch (heart): when the adrenal glands are overworked, the body becomes too stressed out, people can have insomnia and forgetfulness, heart palpitation, shortness of breath, even chest pain, too.

Kidney meridian also serves to have power and strength. People's strength or "life essence" comes from the kidneys, that is, from the waist, which is the house of the kidneys. A strong back and waist shows strong kidney function. If the kidneys are deficient, the person will have weak back, chronic back pain or be hunched over, which is a sign of serious weakness of the kidney Qi; protecting the heart will also be weakened.

Creativity. The kidney essence governs birth, embodied in sperm and eggs, which can create a new life. Only the kidney essence can create life in all the organs.

Storing essence. The essence can fill up the spinal cord and brain when kidney essence is sufficient and the transformation function is strong. This strengthens the person's creativity, quick-wit and ingeniousness, provides energy and repels fear. Fear is a negative emotion of the kidney, too much fear can weaken our kidney. Fear can cause depression and anxiety, so deep depression and anxiety is linked to the lack of kidney Yang Qi and essence, which can also cause brain sluggishness and mental retardation.

Storing essence consolidates one's own life, creates new life allowing one's genes to be better passed on. In this regard, animals should do better than people. Because animals follow simple principles, and humans follow complex principles. For example, a lion must be a lion king after battle. This lion king must be the strongest in wisdom and physical strength. It will have all the smart and beautiful female lions, the good genes will be passed on. But people are much more complicated in this regard. People can marry people with low vitality or low physical ability for money, etc., which leads to the diversity of human nature and physical ability.

Modern times pose many threats: pollution, chemicals, radiation, toxins, life stress, etc. These challenges pose serious problems of infertility. Because gene transmission is the most selfish and instinctive manifestation of all things in the world. I am worried the decline of human creativity will bring a huge crisis to the race.

Governs water. The purpose of heart fire should shine down like the sun. Kidney water must have the ability of transpiration and rise. In this way, there will be the intersection of steam, transformation and metabolism. Yang steams Yin water becoming Qi vapor.

Controls reception of Qi. Kidney holds down Qi sent by lung to prevent congestion. Asthma is a sign of a weakened kidney.

Kidney is the life gate, the root of original Qi - Yuan Qi - prenatal Qi, source of fire -Yang Qi- for all internal organs and function. Strong constitution comes with a strong Yuan Qi. Any chronic disease will weaken the kidney.

Kidney controls bowel movements and urine.

Main indications

Acupuncture points in this meridian are used for gynecological, genital, kidney, lung, and pharynx (throat) diseases. They are also indicated for symptoms associated with the pathway of the meridian.

Symptoms

Disharmony of Kidney Meridian can manifest as asthma, wheezing, coughing, blood in phlegm because the kidneys "grasp the Qi." Asthma and Blood in phlegm are kidney problems, white phlegm and yellow phlegm are lung disease, which means lung has infection.

Edema (swelling), constipation, diarrhea, urination problems as the kidney controls bowel movements and urination.

Pharynx (throat) is located along the meridian's pathway, the throat area problems can indicate a problem with the kidney meridian.

Dry mouth and tongue are associated as saliva is kidney fluid and the kidney meridian relies on the tongue.

The upward fumigation of kidney fluid depends entirely on kidney Yang, and when kidney Yang is deficient, saliva does not rise. The mouth and tongue are dry.

Impotency is related as reproductive energy comes from the kidney. Low sexual performance is kidney energy deficient. No morning erection, lifting is not firm and cannot last. The sperm quality is poor.

Prostate problems such as enlargement and frequent urination. Now, surgery is often used to treat this disease. There was no surgery in ancient times, so ancient healers focused on health preservation methods. For example: gently hold scrotum every night when you sleep, which is referred to as nourishing the outer kidney. Another method is to stand on your toes when you pee, close your mouth, clench your teeth, no talking, and concentrate on peeing. Pee one third at a time, hold for six seconds, then pee another one third, hold for 6 seconds, then finish.

Immune deficiency.

Poor memory or an inability to think clearly.

Insomnia and forgetfulness- the kidneys protect the heart and if they are too stressed out, adrenal glands overworked, people suffer from insomnia and forgetfulness.

Chronic back pain is related to the loss of kidney essence. A large loss of kidney essence can make the back crooked and cause you to hunch over.

Short attention span can also indicate a kidney meridian imbalance. Kidney spirit is ambition or "Zhi." If the kidney spirit is insufficient, the person lacks concentration, takes a short-term view and has a hard time completing tasks.

High blood pressure. Kidney water is the source of liver essence. If the kidney essence is insufficient, the liver Yang will become hyperactive, both diastolic and systolic blood pressure can be high.

Lost appetite- you might feel very hungry, but don't want to eat because kidney meridians are blocked.

Dark face, haggard, without luster. This is the manifestation of kidney disease on the face.

Jaundice: Western medicine believes that jaundice is caused by increased serum bilirubin concentration due to bilirubin metabolism disorders. Clinically, the sclera, mucous membranes, skin and other tissues are stained yellow. In TCM, jaundice is considered to be a disease of the liver and spleen. In order to expel jaundice, the kidney must have a strong diuretic function. If the kidney is deficient, there is no source of jaundice.

Worry, heartache are complications. It is caused by the heart and kidney intersection of steam and transformation is poor. The fire of the heart goes down, and the warm water of the kidneys goes up into clouds and mist, which is the best state of life. If there is no warm kidney water, Qi is stagnant and can create worry. Blood deficiency can lead to heartache.

Muscle atrophy, limbs cold. People are tired, like lying down and don't even have the energy to sit. Strength comes from the kidneys, and if the lungs and kidneys are deficient, people can feel particularly lazy.

Hot and burning feet. The kidney meridian goes under the foot, from the little toe to the Kidney 1, and then to the heel. All problems under the feet are from the kidneys.

Inside of the calf pain can be related to the kidneys and the bladder. Don't underestimate the problem of the calf. Aging starts from the calf and legs. Pain and stiffness of the calf are also related to the great decline of the Yang Qi of the bladder meridian. The midline back of the leg runs through the bladder meridian, the kidney meridian, the liver meridian and the spleen meridian on the inner side, the stomach meridian in the front and the gall-bladder meridian on the outer side. Bladder meridian Qi deficiency is Yang Qi deficiency, kidney meridian deficiency is Yin essence deficiency, so the calf is a very important health indicator of life. Massaging it regularly will delay the aging too.

Goosebumps. When people are frightened or suddenly encounter cold wind, they will get goosebumps. The kidney and the bladder are on the outside and inside and the kidney controls trembling, and the bladder controls the body surface. When people are frightened, the kidney Qi is restrained and the bladder is in a hurry to rescue, the skin becomes corn-like. Sudden encounter with cold wind means the surface is cold, the kidney comes out to save the body surface, and the person trembles. This is the same as menstruation, if only blood is sufficient, without the promotion of Yang, menstruation will still have problems. From the mutual assistance and interaction of body organs, we can understand the mutual assistance and interaction of people, so as to understand why we should be grateful. If there is no proper help from others, our life will not be perfect.

In fact, nourishing the kidney means warming and raising the yang, drinking more warm soups, eating beans, sleeping more and talking less. Avoid toxins and chemicals, indulgence, anger, worry, and sleeping late. Avoid emotional ups and downs.

Absolutely relaxing mentally. When the mind is relaxed, the kidneys are nourished, because the kidneys dominate fear, and when worried or tense the kidneys are damaged.

Need not only to relax the mind, but also to exercise. Go out the door and get a sun bath to generate Yang energy in the body, which can dispel dampness and ward off cold.

Acupoints

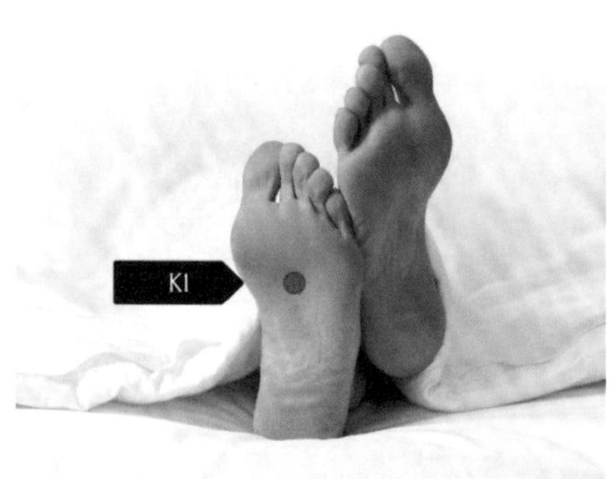

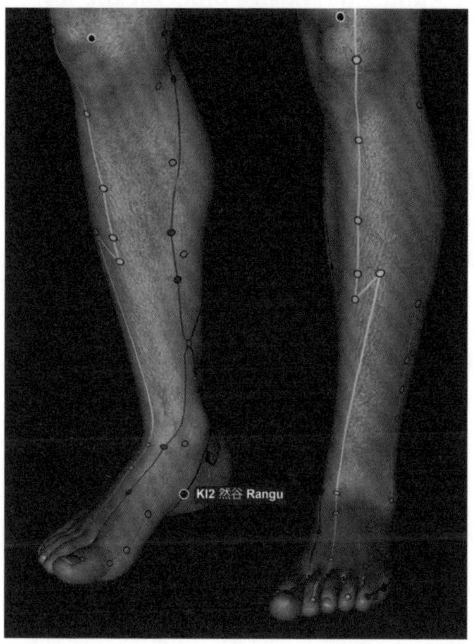

K 1: YONG QUAN (GUSHING SPRING)

Name: Gushing Spring, Jing well points channel of the kidney channel is its first point. A source of water, energy and vibrancy. The name of this point means that the kidney water flows out of the body from here.

Location: On the sole of the foot, in the depression when the foot is in plantar flexion, approximately one third from the base of the second toe, or two thirds from the back of the heel.

Indication: syncope, heat stroke, epilepsy, pediatric convulsions and other emergencies and mental illnesses; in addition, it also treats headache, dizziness; hemoptysis, sore throat; dysuria, constipation; foot heart heat. In modern times, it is commonly used in the treatment of shock, hypertension, insomnia, hysteria, epilepsy, infantile convulsions, nervous headache, enuresis, urinary retention, etc. It is one of the first-aid points.

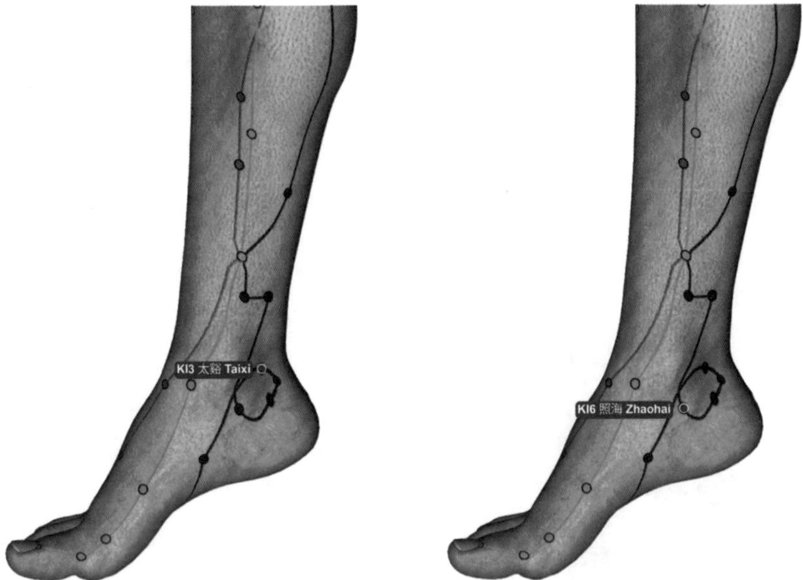

There are also several important kidney meridian points on the feet and inside of the ankle area.

For example, Kidney 2 Ran Gu acupoint is used with Bladder 57 Cheng Shan to treat tendons, and Kidney 3 Tai Xi is used to treat fever, anxiety, cold feet, and profuse sweating. Kidney 6 Zhao Hai point is mainly used for dry throat, epilepsy, insomnia, reclining, panic and restlessness, red eyes, swelling and pain, irregular menstruation, dysmenorrhea, vaginal discharge, vaginal itching, hernia, frequent urination, insomnia, athlete's foot and so on. When you have nothing to do, rub the acupuncture points on your feet well to prevent aging.

Miscellaneous bits:

Element: Water
Direction: North
Season: Winter
Climate: Cold
Cultivation: Hibernate

Sense Organ: Ears
Sense: Hearing
Tissue: Bones
Positive Emotion: Gentleness
Negative Emotion: Fear
Flavor: Salty
Color: Black
Sound: Groaning
Smell: Putrid
Time: 5 p.m. – 7 p.m.
Opposite: Large Intestine
Yin/Yang: Yin
Flow Direction: Up
Origin/Ending: Foot to Chest
Number of Acupoints: 27 on one side of the body, total 54.

Kidney Meditation

Make yourself comfortable… I would like you to gently close your eyes and focus your attention onto the sound of my voice...

As you listen now, I would like you to become aware of your body and tune into your breath...

I want you to give yourself permission to let go… to allow yourself to feel completely relaxed… I wonder if you could take a nice deep breath in, and as you release the breath slowly, let go of all the tension in those muscles around your body.

Give yourself permission to enjoy all the sensations of a deep breath in and then, exhale out all the tensions as you relax...

Short pause.

Let's go on a sacred meditative journey… a journey of transformation… and to understand transformation…

At this moment it is as though you haven't a care in the world - nobody wants anything - nobody needs anything - there is absolutely nothing at all for you to do except relax and let go - and just enjoy the feelings that are being generated within you right now…

You're beginning to realize that any worrying that you've been doing over the past few years hasn't done any good at all ... Life is a series of ups and downs and we have to experience the lows to really appreciate the highs and the middle ground… but when things went wrong in the past you worried until you made yourself ill… and did it do any good?

Ask yourself - does worrying change or improve anything for you? Worry creates stress… worry creates lines on the brow… worry lowers kidney Qi… nobody really likes a worrier because it can make them worry as well… because just like laughter… worry is contagious.

So you decide right now, here in meditation… that you're going to react more positively in the future… instead of worrying your life away you'll take life's ups and downs in stride and remain calm, cool and collected… and most importantly confident ... just remember the four C's - calm, cool, collected and confident… that's you.

There may have been times when you tried to sleep and all life's problems went round and round in your head… that happens a lot to worriers…both are related to kidney imbalance… your mind is still trying to sort things out… and niggles at the back of the mind tend to come forward when we're close to sleep ...

If that's happened to you… don't worry… simply remember the four C's and remain calm, cool, collected and confident ... You remain calm because there's no point in worrying… that won't resolve a thing… you stay cool… everyone wants to be cool… your thoughts are collected - there in your mind - and you're confident that your subconscious mind will find a solution if there's one to be found...

And because you trust yourself - you find that it's easy to drift off somewhere nice before going to sleep. Because you know that any problems in your mind - can be resolved at night in your sleep... that is the power of the subconscious…

So drift away now - to a special place - and leave all those worries and cares behind - you can put them in a drawer or a cupboard - ready to be dealt with at a more appropriate time - or you can send them away on a big black cloud - that cloud that's been hovering over you - send your worries up there - and bring a gust of wind to blow them away - just blow them away... now…

Because right now you're just enjoying these wonderful feelings of calm tranquility - and I wonder if you can see or sense a beautiful stairway in your mind? A stairway with hundreds of steps - going down and down to a beautiful place - and you can begin to descend - gently downwards - going deeper and deeper into meditative rest - deeper and deeper - down and down - and as you go down you may notice - beautiful colors or it may just be comfortably dark and reassuring...

You may notice a beautiful fragrance - that could remind you of something from your past - notice it now - perhaps a special person's perfume or a childhood smell that you loved - can you notice it now?

And as you go deeper down - you decide once and for all that worrying doesn't do any good. From now on you always remember the four Cs - calm, cool, collected and confident - and that makes you feel good - you're in complete control of your mind - your body and your health.

Just enjoy these wonderful feelings - as you reach the bottom of the stairway and looking around - see the beautiful scene that meets your eyes. Just enjoy being here - in your special place - and notice how this place becomes now - a part of you - a wonderful place where you can visit again whenever you wish - all with the power of your mind...

Pause

And as you continue to relish in your special place, let your mind drift to the magic of the meridians and how they work like a network system, transporting and distributing Qi and blood ... how the meridians link up organs, limbs, joints, bones, tendons, tissues and skin, and provide communication between the body interior and exterior, through a healthy meridian system...

Marvel at the magic of how Qi and blood successfully warm and nourish different organs and tissues, and maintain normal metabolic activities...

Understand that meridians are essential in supporting the flow of nutritive Qi inside the blood vessels and flow of protective Qi around them ... they strengthen the body's immunity, protect against external pernicious influences and assist in regulating Yin and Yang ...

Know that kidney is known as the "Minister of Power." It is tasked with storing the prenatal energy as well as the essential vital energy for life.

Also known as the "mansion of fire and water," and the "residence of yin and yang," the kidney also works at regulating the brain and plays an important role in the formation of memories and rationality.

Returning now to your breath, you know that each gentle out-breath can lead to more and more relaxation...

Paying attention to your breathing can help you relax even more...

Know that strength or "life essence" comes from the kidneys, that is, from the waist, which is the house of the kidneys… A strong back and waist shows strong kidney function ... guard against kidneys deficiency to avoid a weak back, chronic back pain hunching over…

Understand that from 5 pm to 7 pm, meridian Qi mainly flows through the Kidney meridian, this is the best time to eat your dinner and restore your energy ... know that the kidneys store energy reserves ... be sure to put yourself first when it comes to your energy ...

Continue to sit back, relaxed, breathing evenly and slowly, calmly and regularly…

There is no time, but now, there is no place but here and right now and right here, you are safe, supported and relaxed ... sooner or later, you'll find yourself wondering about going into an even deeper state of relaxation, and you may do that suddenly or gradually...

As you do this, you feel your body becoming heavier and heavier as every muscle in your body begins to let go as you sink deeper – and deeper – into this wonderful feeling of peace and tranquility...

Allow for the kidney to store your essence ... this essence can fill up the spinal cord and brain when kidney essence is sufficient and the transformation function is strong ... know that this will strengthen your creativity, quicken your wit and ingeniousness… provide energy and repel fear ...

Understand that fear is a negative emotion of the kidney, too much fear can weaken our kidney ... fear can cause depression and anxiety… deep depression and anxiety are linked to the lack of kidney yang Qi and essence… this imbalance can also cause brain sluggishness and mental retardation....

Understand fear and embrace it ... fear exists to keep us safe ... it is not inherently bad or good but a tool we can use to make better decisions ... fear isn't designed to keep us inactive, but to help us act in ways that generate the results we need and want ... embrace fear as instruction and let it inform your actions, but not control them ... this will strengthen kidney Qi

Visualize balanced transformation throughout your body, your meridians and especially your kidney meridian…

Know that as yin and yang continuously adjust to one another and transform into one another there is a never-ending dance of harmonization… when the organs have sufficient yang qi normal metabolism follows, which promotes qi transformation ... if the kidney is full of qi, you are likely to be sharp, energetic and fearless ...

Embrace that if we live a risk-averse existence because of fear, we also live a joy-averse existence ... the life you live depends on the choices you make and the sometimes calculated risks you take ... they are the very ingredients in the recipe called happiness ... overcoming fears means that great otherwise unforeseen opportunities might come your way… perhaps a new job, a new relationship or a new opportunity for growth ... overcoming fears forces us to learn and embracing risk-taking also helps you to overcome a fear of failure ... all of which strengthen your kidney Qi…

Set your intention to grow awareness of your power of meridian balance and harmony and understand that you can resist being carried along on a current not of your own making… resist blaming external forces for anything in your life… instead shaping your experience by setting your intention to achieve what you want and by extension affect your outer world experience…

Accept that the key to a harmonious mind is to be able to think clearly and to be transparent with your heart… which guards against stress between the brain and heart ... understanding that you can make yourself sick by fretting about problems ....

Breathe deeply and align your brain and heart to work through issues ... Prepare for making the unconscious conscious through meditation, which will result in balanced meridians, enhanced focus, increased emotional intelligence, greater mental strength, improved physical health, healthy relationships and ultimately to self-realization...

Give yourself permission to embrace a new awareness of your power to create reality through the balancing of your meridians, through meditation and how this awareness will prepare you to live unconditionally...

notice the happiness you feel inside knowing how powerful meridian balance is and how connected to humanity you are...notice how this connection fills you with an elevated vibration... and how an elevated vibration can expand the visible spectrums of your senses...

Now just breathe and be with yourself and let the waves of your breathing be with you...

CHAPTER NINE

Pericardium Meridian

Characteristics

Known in TCM as the "Heart Protector" or "Circulation-Sex" Meridian, the pericardium is associated with the FIRE element and the HEART.

The pericardium protects the heart from emotional trauma, constricts the chest to protect the heart, and helps to express the joy of the heart. While not an organ, the pericardium does correspond to an actual part of the body. The pericardium is a protective sack encircling the heart.

From seven pm to nine pm, meridian Qi mainly flows through the pericardium meridian. This is the best time to get a massage, have sex and to conceive.

Socialize.

Have fun!

The pericardium meridian is a unique concept in TCM, it is known as the Ambassador to the Emperor (heart), and from it joy and happiness derives. The pericardium is a protective sack encircling the heart. Its protection extends beyond the physical including the mental, emotional, and spiritual.

It is responsible for regulating circulation of the blood. The pericardium meridian also links the emotional feelings of love with the physical act of sex. And, it assists the triple warmer with its functions. It is one of the two principal meridians not associated with a major organ, the other being the Triple warmer. It can be seen as both a bizarre and a unique system.

The pericardium is the internal energy that promotes the movement and transformation of the triple warmer. The reason why the organs do not sag is because of the energy of the triple warmer, but where does the energy of the triple warmer come from? The pericardium. We will discuss triple warmer more in the next chapter.

The pericardium and triple warmer are negatively affected differently. The pericardium suffers as a meridian, the triple warmer suffers as Qi; Qi is in the meridians so these two meridians are interconnected like a couple. The triple warmer is the vitality and the beginning of the Yang Qi. Its Qi is fresh and agile, without obstructions, and it permeates the whole body. His wife is the pericardium, and is happy and joyful. Therefore, they are like the bride and groom. That is to say, when the wife is happy, the husband is happy too. Much like life itself! The triple warmer and the pericardium system are a unique system of the human body, from which the happiness of life and the transparency of life emerge.

This symbiotic relationship, invisible and intangible as they may seem, are very important to life itself in equally unseen ways.

The pericardium, in Western medicine, refers to the membranous sack covering the surface of the heart and wrapped around the heart and the roots of the great blood vessels that go in and out of the heart. There is a cavity between the visceral and wall layers, called the pericardial cavity. The pericardium has a protective effect on the heart, preventing surrounding infections from spreading to the heart; limiting the expansion of the heart and preventing the rapid rupture of the heart when intracardiac pressure rises. The most common symptom is pericardial effusion. The clinical manifestation is mainly dull chest pain. Generally, pericardiocentesis is used to relieve the symptoms caused by the compression of surrounding organs. Note that this is just a relief, not a cure. In traditional Chinese medicine, it is generally called palpitations or water heart disease. Ling Gui Zhu Gan herb decoction is known to have a miraculous effect.

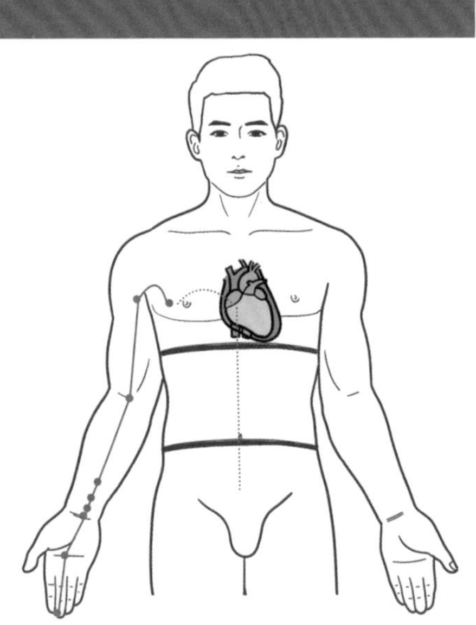

Primary Pathway

The pericardium meridian starts from the chest, leaves the pericardium and runs downwards through the diaphragm to connect with the triple warmer.

A branch rising from the chest emerges from the lower chest region and travels upwards to the axilla (armpit).

From the medial aspect of the upper arm, it makes its way down between the lung and heart channels, until it reaches the elbow crease.

It then runs down the forearm and enters the palm ending at the tip of the middle finger.

Another short branch splits off from the palm to connect with the triple burner meridian at the end of the ring finger.

The kidney meridian and the pericardium meridian are connected in the chest. This is the endless loop of the meridians.

Main Indication

Acupuncture points in this meridian are used for heart, chest, and peptic diseases as well as mental illness. They are also indicated for symptoms manifested along the meridian's pathway.

Imbalances can cause problems with the heart, chest, stomach, and mind. Imbalances with the pericardium meridian are often caused by extreme, sustained outbursts of emotion.

The pericardium in TCM is different from Western medicine, but the heart protection function is the same. And in TCM, an ***important aspect of the pericardium meridian is that it is related to Danzhong.***

Danzhong (Ren 17)

It is located in the middle of the two breasts where the pericardium meridian Qi gathers, comes out and collects. Danzhong can not only cure pericardium diseases, but also dredge the Qi of the whole body.

The thymus gland corresponds to the Danzhong in Chinese medicine. The thymus gland produces T cells, which have a role in preventing cancer. And TCM says that joy comes out of Danzhong, which shows that joy prevents cancer. In other words, unhappiness and pain are the root cause of disease and even cancer.

Small fetuses have extremely large red thymus glands, but after birth, the thymus glands shrink rapidly. This is like a person's life. The fastest growing period is the fetal period. From the fertilized egg to birth, it takes ten months for a small fetus to complete hundreds of thousands of years of human evolution.

Without joy, the meridians will not be smooth, the Qi and blood will not be healthy, and life will not grow. After birth, all internal organs grow. Only the thymus gland rapidly atrophies, which means that one is born into death.

We always think that we are born to be strong, but in terms of the ultimate destination of life we are actually on the road to decay from the very beginning and the end point of life is inevitable death.

The source of disease is related. If the Danzhong is damaged, the T cells will be damaged, there will be no power to resist illness and people will become seriously ill.

Real happiness is not to laugh three times a day, but to find joy within Dharma (although laughter can be good). This kind of Dharma bliss comes from awakening spiritually to life, a simple life, a peaceful mind, a reserve of Qi and essence, unattached to material desires, without emotional disturbance, happiness independent from the quality of foreign objects or material gains and losses.

It is not your brain that is asking for happiness. It is your body that is actually asking you to be happy. Eating well, sleeping well, and having a normal sex life must be your life's underlying premise. Therefore, the joy of the pericardium is first and foremost the joy of our nature.

So, when you are angry, it has more to do with you not understanding your life, not understanding human nature.

What is the first step to being happy? Remove yourself from people and situations that annoy you. If you can't even do this step, how can you be happy?

Many of my patients frequently ask me when the disease will heal. The first thing to look for is when you will be happy, once you are happy Qi, meridians and blood will be smooth and then disease can be eliminated.

Another function of Danzhong is to block evil spirits. The ancients did not know what T cells were, but they knew that Danzhong could block evil Qi, and blocking evil Qi was blocking cancer cells. Western medicine says that T cells are produced here, which can prevent cancer. As long as T cells are abundant, people will not have cancer. When people get old, the thymus shrinks even more, so cancer is an aging disease. When a young person gets cancer, it means that they are aging fast. Danzhong is negatively affected by suffering and holding back diminishes it.

So how do you usually strengthen the function of Danzhong?

You massage the Danzhong. If you feel that your hand is not strong enough, you can scrape with a Jade scraper.

Diseases, including cancer cells, are actually equivalent to seeds. When people get old, their Qi and blood decline, and their cells are inactive. There may be cancer cells in everyone's body, that is, things that grow disorderly or mutate.

But whether the seeds germinate or not is related to the soil and the environment of life. If you are angry and depressed, the surrounding environment will be bad, and bad seeds may germinate.

Western medicine first regarded cancer as a mission, but now it is found that the cure rate is not high, and the misdiagnosis rate is very high. Therefore, by killing the seeds, it is better to change the environment; instead of killing, it is better to reconcile, and it is better to prolong life.

Where does cancer metastasize? The triple warmer meridian. It is the channel, the visible and the invisible all transferred through this channel.

That pericardium should be the scavenger on this passage. Without this minister, the triple warmer channel would be filthy and unclear.

The unhappiness of the pericardium will also block the triple warmer channel. So if you want to avoid cancer, you have to work hard on joy, happiness and body meridians.

Symptoms

Heart issues, stroke, hypertension, breast lumps.

Rage, depression, anxiety, worry which is not only associated with the pericardium, but also associated with the lung, spleen and kidney meridians.

All kinds of awkwardness and discomfort in the arms and elbows, even arm cramps.

Inflammation of the lymph nodes.

The chest and ribs feeling of fullness.

Hot palms. The hot palm is the fire of the heart, and the hot feet is the excess of the kidney Yang. Babies are pure Yang bodies, and sometimes they may be like this, it's not a disease.

Red or pale face, eyes yellow, laughs a lot, there are also early signs of heart attack, people might not know.

The expression of heart disease on the complexion, one is pale complexion, which is a disease that has been severely damaged by heart blood, and the other is red complexion, ochre red, which is usually a heart disease associated with high blood pressure.

Acupoints

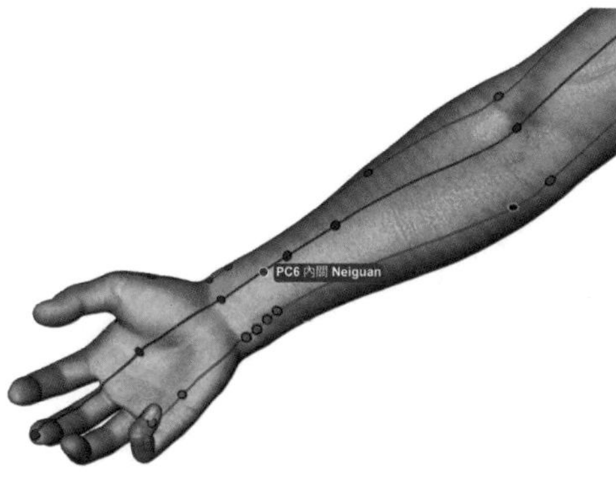

P 6: NEI GUAN (INNER BORDER GATE)

Name: Inner Border Gate, can either bring Qi inside or clear things that are in or attempting to go into the interior. Allows the Heart to regulate Boundaries
Location: two inches above the wrist crease, the place where two tendons seem to be sandwiched is Neiguan.
Indication: An emergency acupoint for heart disease. It should be massaged frequently, which is effective for heartache, palpitations, chest tightness, and chest pain. Commonly used in the treatment of heart pain, angina pectoris, myocarditis, arrhythmia, gastritis, hysteria and nausea and so on.
Technique and notes: Massage

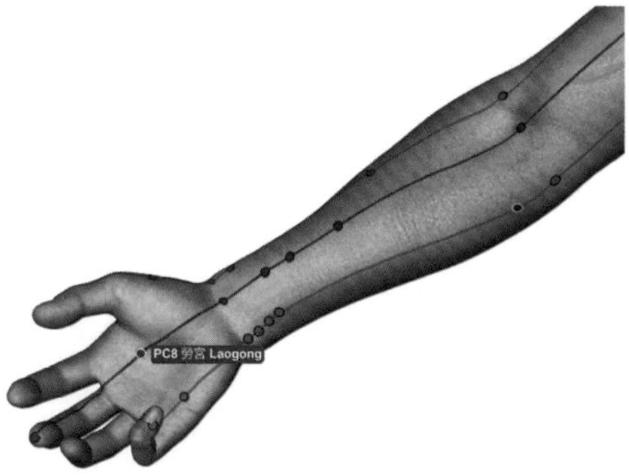

P 8 LAO GONG (PALACE OF LABOR)

Name: Palace of Labor, the reason why Laogong is called Laogong is because it is the hardest acupoint in our body. It can clear heart heat, purify liver fire, and reassure the mind.
Location: When the fist is clenched, the point is just below the tip of the middle finger, on the crease between the second and third metacarpal bones.
Indication: It can be used to treat insomnia and neurasthenia. Tongue ulcers, epilepsy. Sweaty palms and high blood pressure.

Pressing the Laogong acupoint can also treat sudden rise in blood pressure. Hypertensive patients will sharply increase their blood pressure

due to anger or excitement. At this time, they can press the Laogong point, and then press each fingertip one by one. When pressing, keep calm and breathe evenly. Blood pressure that suddenly rises after compressions can be relieved.
Technique and note: Massage.

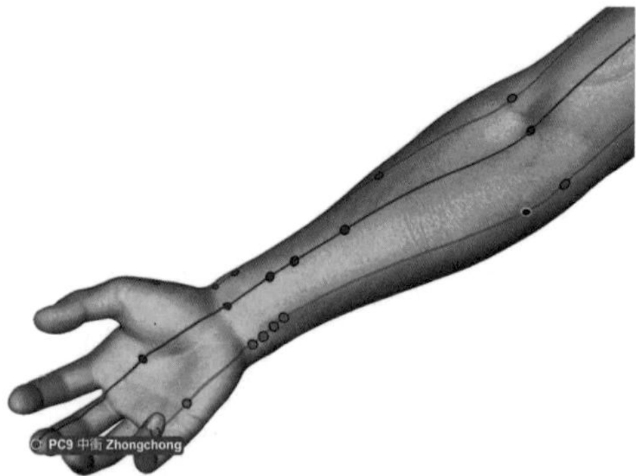

P 9 ZHONG CHONG (CENTRAL HUB)

Name: Central Hub, here is where pericardium has a direct connection with Chong, travels along the middle path, and rushes straight to the end of the middle finger, hence the name Zhong Chong.
Location: In the center area on the tip of the middle finger.
Indications: Stroke, coma, tongue suffocation, heat stroke, fainting, convulsions in children, fever, swelling and pain under the tongue, and night crying in children.
Technique and Notes: Massage or prick bleeding, or moxibustion with moxa sticks for one to three minutes, you can also snap your fingers dredging the pericardium.

Miscellaneous bits:

There are just nine acupoints in the pericardium meridian. The most important are Neiguan and Zhongchong. It is important to note here that Danzhong is not the acupoint of the pericardium, but of the Ren meridian. The relationship between Danzhong and the pericardium is actually the relationship between the Ren channel and the pericardium; the pericardium is related to the congenital meridians.
Element: Fire
Direction: South

Season: Summer
Climate: Heat
Sense Organ: Tongue
Sense: Touch
Tissue: Vessels
Positive Emotion: Joy
Negative Emotion: Arrogance
Flavor: Bitter; Color: Purple Red
Sound: Laughter
Smell: Scorched
Time: 7 p.m. - 9 p.m.
Opposite: Stomach
Yin/Yang: Yin
Flow Direction: Up
Origin/Ending: Chest to Hand
Number of Acupoints: 9 on one side of the body, total 18.

Pericardium Meditation

Take three slow, deep breaths and prepare yourself for a meditative journey…

Make yourself comfortable… and focus your attention onto the sound of my voice...

As you listen now, I would like you to become aware of your body and tune into your breath...

Short pause.

And as you focus your mind on the sound of my voice, I would like you to relax all the muscles in your body - and if you notice any tension anywhere in your body - just let it go - let it go completely - and relax even deeper.

As you begin to check those muscles, relaxing each and every one, just feel and experience heaviness in those eyelids - a comfortable, heavy feeling that begins to weigh your lids down.

And all the while you are letting go of tension, listening to the sound of my voice and concentrating on that heavy, comfortable feeling in and around your eyes...

And as those eyes become heavier and more relaxed - so they begin blinking more and more - perhaps even feeling a little watery - and that's alright - because whenever you wish to close those eyes - you can do so - and allow them to remain closed - as you continue listening to the sound of my voice.

Understand that the pericardium is the Ambassador to the Emperor and protects the heart from emotional trauma, constricts the chest to protect the heart, and helps to express the joy of the heart...

Allow yourself to see that your key to achieving your dreams and desires lies in your understanding that you are the keeper of your joy and happiness, the key to knowing yourself and what you want and why, which in turn has the capacity to deliver the best you…

Become aware of the fact that you cannot control the outer world, understand that control of the outer world is an illusion...

Bring your awareness to the fact that your joy and your happiness are your responsibility…gratitude, meditation, quiet stillness, are the gateways to happiness and joy… know that mastering this recognition places you into the position that will allow you to create your reality; with practice, any mindstate can be brought to happiness in meditation… joy can be embraced through the understanding of your power to create it…

Let your mind drift to the magic of the meridians and how they work like a network system, transporting and distributing Qi and blood ... how the meridians link up organs, limbs, joints, bones, tendons, tissues and skin, and provide communication between the body interior and exterior, through a healthy meridian system...

Marvel at the magic of how Qi and blood successfully warm and nourish different organs and tissues, and maintain normal metabolic activities...

Understand that meridians are essential in supporting the flow of nutritive Qi inside the blood vessels and flow of protective Qi around them ... they strengthen the body's immunity, protect against external pernicious influences and assist in regulating Yin and Yang ...

Give yourself permission to dive deeply in joy… give yourself permission to believe that if you can hold happiness in your mind, you can hold it in your life… to recognize that you are joyful and happy because you want to be, you can feel connected in positive and loving thoughts for yourself and for others…

Create an awareness of your ability to live in joy, to create your own happiness no matter what is going on around you… understand and nurture the fact that we can always, no matter the state of the world around us, bring ourselves into joy and happiness connecting us with our wholeness; we can direct our thoughts to love, kindness, gratitude and forgiveness… to joy, happiness and the details of our dreams…

Know that the pericardium meridian is responsible for regulating circulation of the blood. The pericardium meridian also links the emotional feelings of love with the physical act of sex...

Embrace that real happiness is not to laugh three times a day, but to find joy within Dharma (although laughter can be good) ... this kind of Dharma bliss comes from awakening spiritually to life… a simple life… a peaceful mind… a reserve of Qi and essence… unattached to material desires… without emotional disturbance… happiness independent from the quality of foreign objects or material gains and losses...

Feel how your acceptance of your permanent possession of joy empowers you to alter your mindstate; how your joy and happiness are inseparable and can provide the opportunity to not only shift from wherever you are to love and kindness, but also to project that love and kindness to others…

Embrace the opportunity to disengage from negative emotions: anger, jealousy, insecurities, and sadness merely by realizing that you possess joy and happiness and in your happy joy, connected to the joy of the human tribe…

Find your power in your joy and the spiritual awakening that it brings; fully understand that with practice, living in joy and creating our own happiness can become the process for understanding and accepting your life purpose ... learning to observe yourself and your joy as the first step toward moving away from powerless states of mind and a belief that external forces control you… toward an empowered "joyful, happy state…. "

Visualize yourself in your joyful happiness as an inoculation against any and all external conditions and influences, visualize joy as the avenue to self-realization through the act of living a joyful, happy life…

Understand that it is not your brain that is asking for happiness ... it is your body that is actually asking you to be happy ... eating well, sleeping well, and having a normal sex life must be your life's underlying premise ... Therefore, the joy of the pericardium is first and foremost the joy of our nature ...

See yourself grounded, balanced and clear on your growing sense of joy… see the complete acceptance of your joy being the foundation for the ability to bring your self-awareness to who you are and who you want to be- regardless of where you may have started from ... and from there, deliberately achieving your dreams and your happiness… and keeping you pericardium meridian healthy, which in turn keeps your heart and other meridians smooth, balanced and healthy, warding off disease…

Understand that awareness of your joy is the key to health, wealth and happiness ... when we understand that we are in control of our joy and find it sometimes the smallest of joyful things, we engage the universe in giving us what we want…

Give yourself permission to practice resting in an energetic field of pure joy… building inner happiness...

Stay away from expectations or judgmental attitudes of others… understand that joy is your pathway to cultivate your truest and highest goals… it is through this awareness of your own everlasting joy that we can also nurture love, kindness, and forgiveness for self and others.…

Breathe in these changes as you understand that the recognition of your joy can be immediate; and your understanding of just how happy you are can be molded over a course of ongoing experiences… know that these experiences will help you create and define your human connection ...

Notice the sensations and breathe… inhale and exhale…

Understand that you, your joy and happiness, are all far more interesting than any low vibrational events currently circulating on the news or masquerading as entertainment… and as you do, your thoughts will become filled with meaning- the moment you think they are. And joy is always within your reach....

Draw your awareness right now to the anticipation of entering the world of pure potential through accepting your joy... embrace the understanding pouring into your being through waves of acceptance and awareness...

Give yourself permission for a new awareness of your joy, and how this awareness will prepare you to live fully...Breathe deeply and align your brain and heart to work through issues ... Prepare for making the unconscious conscious through meditation, which will result in balanced meridians, enhanced focus, increased emotional intelligence, greater mental strength, improved physical health, healthy relationships and ultimately to self-realization...

Give yourself permission to embrace a new awareness of your power to create reality through the balancing of your meridians, through meditation and how this awareness will prepare you to live unconditionally...

notice the happiness you feel inside knowing how powerful meridian balance is and how connected to humanity you are...notice how this connection fills you with an elevated vibration... and how an elevated vibration can expand the visible spectrums of your senses...

Now just breathe and be with yourself and let the waves of your breathing be with you...

CHAPTER TEN

Triple Warmer / San Jiao Meridian

Characteristics

Also known as the triple burner or San Jiao, the triple warmer meridian is unique in that it is not energetically tied to a specific organ in the body.

In fact, this meridian helps to regulate all the organs and energy in the body.

This is why the triple warmer is often referred to as the organ with function, but no form.

From nine pm to eleven pm, meridian Qi mainly flows through the triple warmer meridian. This is the best time to chill out.

Relax.

Don't eat!

The triple warmer is the official in charge of irrigation, metabolic passage of water, Yuan, or original Qi and prenatal Qi.

Water makes up about 70 percent of the human body, so the distribution of this water is very important to the smooth operation of human life.

The triple warmer governs all the Qi of internal organs and meridians: inside and outside, left and right, and upper and lower.

The function is to irrigate the whole body, to adjust and balance the internal and external, to nourish the left and the right and to guide the upper and lower.

From this, it can be seen that the triple warmer is of great significance to the human body.

As noted, the triple warmer is not an actual organ, but it is similar to the thyroid in that it controls the metabolism. It is not strictly limited to the energetic metabolism, though. It is also involved in digestion and waste processing.

It is the channel, the visible and the invisible and everywhere, all revolving around this channel. It's the space between the organs. Just like celestial phenomena, there is space between the sun, moon and stars, and that space is even more significant than the sun, moon and stars.

This "emptiness" in the body controls the internal organs and meridians. How does it govern? The governance relies on Qi. The internal organs do not sag or sway in the thoracic and abdominal cavities because of the Qi of the triple warmer. In short, given the important function of the triple warmer, it can be considered the largest organ of the human body.

As the name suggests, there are three parts to the triple warmer: upper, middle, and lower.

The upper warmer runs from the base of the tongue to the stomach. It controls bodily intake of food, water, and oxygen. The upper warmer energy is like mist, transporting and transforming moisture quickly with no room for condensation. If fluids are condensed it means that the function of the upper warmer has a problem. Emotions like anger affect the upper warmer in actions like holding one's breath.

The middle warmer starts at the stomach and ends at the pyloric valve. It is responsible for digestion and transformation for use by the body. The middle warmer energy is like a maceration chamber where ripening takes place; the ripening can't be too fast or too slow thus transportation and transformation are medium-speed. Too fast and decomposition is incomplete; too slow content rots and deteriorates.

The lower burner then splits, ending at the anus and urinary tract. It handles the elimination of wastes. Lower warmer energy is like a drainage ditch, which refers to the state of rapid transformation of water and liquid which should be collected, eliminated, so that Yin and Yang can communicate.

The connection of the three is: the middle warmer is the root of the upper warmer, the lower warmer is the root of the middle warmer, and the essence of the rapid transformation of the upper warmer is returned to the lower warmer.

In this way, it is the Qi mechanism of the human body, of which the middle warmer is the key point, and it is the source of the human body's Qi and blood. Blockages or imbalance mean that body fluid flow can't function, that is, the Qi can't rise up!

The human omental system (a fold of the peritoneum -the thin tissue that lines the abdomen- that surrounds the stomach and other organs in the abdomen) in Western medicine is similar to the triple warmer, which was discovered two thousand years ago in the Yellow Emperor's Internal Medicine.

The grain of skin and the texture of the subcutaneous flesh also belongs to the triple warmer.

When triple warmer Qi is full and the nutrients are full, the person looks young and the skin is elastic.

When people are old, the triple warmer Yang Qi declines, and nutrients are deficient. The skin is shriveled and sags. Triple warmer suffers from Qi diseases. When Qi is full, the omentum is plump, and life is also fresh and agile.

When the triple warmer Qi has a problem, it is not an ordinary disease and the internal organs may collapse along with it. When the Qi mechanism of the whole body is not smooth, it means congestion, it means freezing and it is connected to the pericardium, which relates to sorrow, and immunity rapidly declines. Cancer cells may appear and metastasize through the triple warmer channel. Therefore, we need to raise our understanding of the triple warmer meridian to a new level.

The triple warmer transports original Qi. The Yuan Qi reaches the internal organs and all parts of the body through the triple warmer. Therefore, the triple warmer is responsible for Qi diseases, and circulate the vital Qi throughout the whole body.

They are the passages of the human body's Qi rising and exiting, and also the place of Qi transformation. Therefore, it is said that the triple warmer has the function of presiding over all Qi and supervising the whole body's Qi movement and Qi transformation.

If the vital Qi is weak and the triple warmer channel does not run smoothly or declines, it will lead to the phenomenon of Qi deficiency in the whole body or in certain parts of the body and its effect is incomparable.

Triple warmer is the house of transmutation. It has the function of imparting water and food essence to Qi, and has the function of transferring dross.

Triple warmer transports water and facilitates the passage of water metabolism. It manages water, dredges water channels, and runs water according to different states of water.

Although the metabolism of water in the human body is completed by the cooperation of the stomach, spleen, lung, kidney, intestine, bladder and other viscera, the rise and fall of water in and out of the human body and the circulation of the whole body can only be achieved through the triple warmer as a channel.

Therefore, the smoothness of the triple warmer waterway not only affects the slow speed of water running, but also inevitably affects the distribution and excretion of water by the viscera.

It can also be said that the operation of water and fluid by the triple warmer is a comprehensive summary of the functions of the spleen, lung, kidney and other organs in charge of water and fluid metabolism.

If the Triple warmer waterway is unfavorable, the functions of the spleen, lungs, kidneys and other viscera to regulate water will be difficult to achieve, resulting in abnormal water metabolism, obstacles to water distribution and excretion, resulting in phlegm, edema and other diseases.

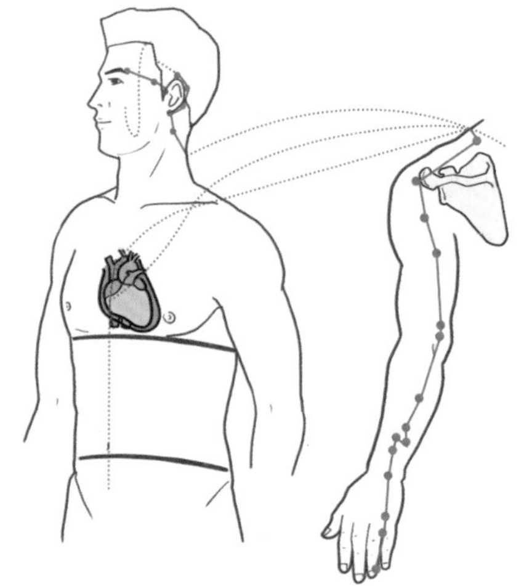

Primary Pathway

The Triple Warmer Meridian begins at the outer tip of the ring finger and goes along the back of the hand, wrist, forearm and upper arm, until it reaches the shoulder region where it branches off.

One branch travels internally into the chest and passes through the pericardium and diaphragm uniting the upper, middle and lower burner.

The other branch runs externally up the side of the neck, circles the ear and face, and finally ends at the outer end of the eyebrow where it connects with the gall bladder meridian.

The pericardium and the triple warmer are external and internal.

The pericardium is the internal power that promotes the movement and transformation of the triple warmer.

Without the power of the pericardium to dredge the ventilator, the movement and transformation of the triple warmer is also powerless.

Main Indication

Acupuncture points in this meridian are recommended for ailments of the ears, eyes, chest, pharynx (throat), and the side of the head as well as certain febrile conditions. They are also indicated for symptoms along this meridian's pathway.

Symptoms

Disharmony of the triple warmer meridian leads to the following symptoms.

Tinnitus, deafness. They are both hard to treat in Western medicine. Anti-inflammatory might be most commonly used to treat; if ineffective, a doctor will tell you to live with it. In my opinion, acute deafness is easier to treat than tinnitus, because tinnitus is basically a deficiency disease, while acute deafness is an acute disease. Acute disease is much easier to treat than chronic. For tinnitus patients, the roaring sound is easier to treat than the low pitching sounds, but if it gets chronic for a long time, it will be difficult to cure. Among them, those with no ringing during the day and aggravated tinnitus at night are Yang deficiency, so in addition to Yin deficiency, anger, cold and other factors, the problem of Yang deficiency should be considered.

Pain in the pharynx (throat), eyes, cheek, back of the ear. Sore throat.

Keratitis, myopia, neurological atrophy, trigeminal neuralgia, facial nerve palsy, etc.

Sweating. This sweating is caused by the failure of the triple warmer to control the waterway. If you sweat too much, sweat profusely, you will definitely kill the Yang.

Abdominal distention, edema (swelling), urinary incontinence, difficulty urinating,

Ache and pain along this meridian's pathway, shoulders, elbows and arms, the little finger and the second finger.

Acupoints

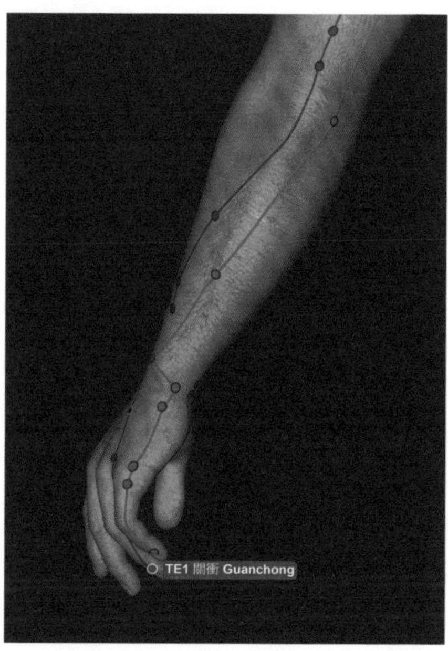

SJ 1 GUAN CHONG (RUSHING GATE)

Name: Rushing Gate/Chong Obstacles, Chong deposits energy into the internal organs. This point assists any obstacle in the dissemination of Yuan Qi. Anything that prevents us from substantiation, having a sense of space, grounding our lives.
Location: on the ulnar end of the ring finger.
Indications: fever, fainting, heat stroke. As well as headache, red eyes, deafness, sore throat and so on.
Technique and notes: massage or bleeding.

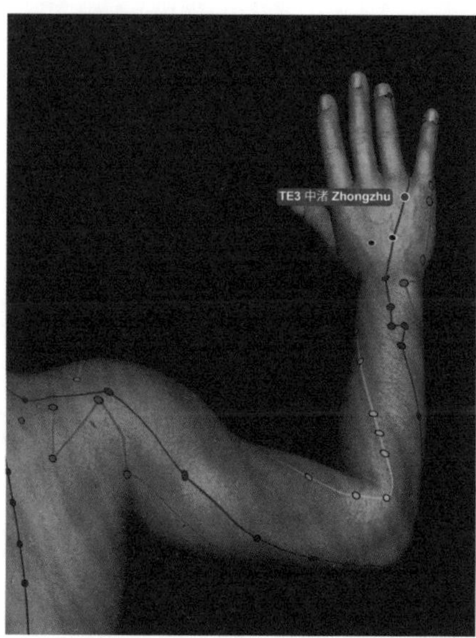

SJ - 3 ZHONG ZHU (CENTRAL ISLET)

Name: Central Islet/City Center, transform Gu Qi to postnatal Qi to use with spleen point.
Location: On the dorsum of the hand, when the fist is clenched, the point is between the fourth and fifth metacarpal bones, in the hollow proximal to the metacarpophalangeal joint.
Indications: headache, tinnitus, deafness, red eyes, sore throat. Fever, diabetes, malaria. Unfavorable
Technique and notes: Massage.

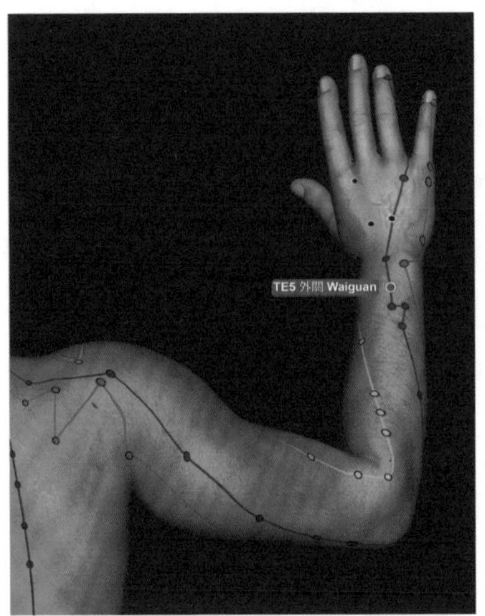

SJ 5 WAI GUAN (OUTER BORDER GATE)

Name: Outer Border Gate, helps to bring things out. Regulate boundaries.

Location: On the forearm, between the radius and ulna, 2 cun (3 fingers) above wrist crease.

Indication: is mainly used for headache, migraine, cheek pain, red eyes and swelling pain, tinnitus, deafness and other head, face and five sense disorders. As well as pain in the hands and five fingers, unable to hold objects, pain in the flanks, pain in the upper limbs, soreness in the elbows, pain in the arms, and intercostal neuralgia.

Technique and notes: Massage

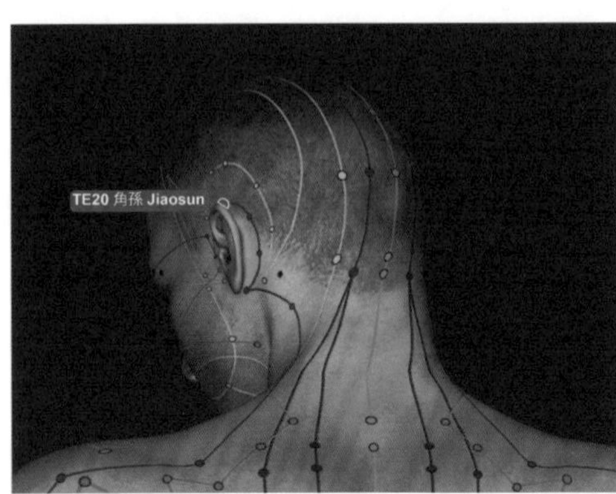

SJ 20 JIAO SUN (ANGLE VERTEX)

Name: Angel Vertex: anatomical location. The angle above the ear.

Location: Directly superior the ear apex, within the hairline. Fold the auricle forward, directly above the tip of the ear and enter the hairline.

Indication: Tinnitus, redness, pain and swelling of ear, ear infection, Pink eyes, swelling of the gum, toothache, eye problem, stiff neck, etc.

Technique: Massage or moxibustion with moxa sticks for 5-10 minutes.

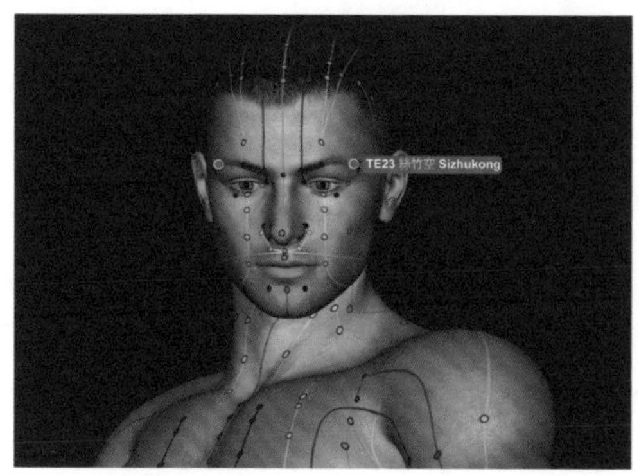

SJ 23: SI ZHU KONG (SILK BAMBOO HOLLOW)

Name: Silk Bamboo Hollow, directs Shen inward. This point is good for those defined by their relationship to others (mom, wife, husband, etc.).
Location: In the depression at the lateral end of the eyebrow
Indication: Headache, redness and pain in eyes, blurry vision, twitching of eyelid, toothache, facial paralysis and epilepsy.
Technique and notes: Massage. Moxibustion is prohibited here.

Miscellaneous bits:

There are 23 points on one side of the Sanjiao meridian, 13 points are on the outer side of the upper arm, and 10 points are distributed on the side head, neck and shoulder. Total 46.
Element: Fire
Direction: South
Season: Summer
Climate: Heat
Cultivation: Growth
Time: 9 p.m. - 11 p.m.
Sense Organ: Tongue
Sense: Touch
Tissue: Vessels
Positive Emotion: Joy
Negative Emotion: Arrogance
Flavor: Bitter
Color: Orange Red
Sound: Laughter
Smell: Scorched

Opposite: Spleen
Yin/Yang: Yang
Flow Direction: Down
Origin/Ending: Hand to Face
Number of Acupoints: 23

Triple Warmer Meditation

Take three slow, deep breaths and prepare yourself for a meditative journey…

Make yourself comfortable… and focus your attention onto the sound of my voice...

As you listen now, I would like you to become aware of your body and tune into your breath...

Short pause.

Now - gently close your eyes and allow yourself to become as comfortable as you possibly can.

Take another nice deep breath - and just exhale - and as you do - give yourself permission to relax.

And each time that you give yourself permission to relax - notice how your body responds - easily - quickly.

And with each moment that passes - you relax just that little bit more - more than a moment ago - realizing, that as we continue - you will hear sounds inside, or outside of the room - but those sounds will only serve to relax you even more - as you listen to my voice - and the sound of the music - these sounds will go with you, wherever your mind wanders - and your mind will wander.

That doesn't matter, because my voice will continue giving you suggestions for relaxation, good feelings, and safe natural healing.

So from this moment on - give yourself permission to go down to your special place.

That special place inside your mind… where everything is perfect for you… you know where that place is, don't you?

Of course, you do… it's the land of your dreams… the place where you are safe, secure, and warm.

And from this moment on… I don't want you to move again until I ask you to… simply follow my suggestions… you could resist, but that's not why you're here, is it?

Of course not… and you realize from this moment on… how much more aware you are… of how relaxed you feel… all of your senses are much more acutely aware - and with each breath you take, you relax more and more… completely relaxed… feeling wonderful.

You experience your thought processes reacting much more calmly… you begin to relax all of your muscles and all of the nerves in your entire body… starting from the top of your head down to the tips of your toes.

You are realizing that you're learning each and every moment how to experience this wonderful feeling of relaxation.

And by learning this method you can use this for yourself… if and when you feel the need… to sleep much easier and to waken much more refreshed.

Realizing that although your conscious mind will drift away - your subconscious hears absolutely everything… and remembers everything perfectly.

And in a moment, I am going to count from 1 to 3… and when I say the number 3… I want you to begin to relax all those little muscles in and around your eyelids… these are the smallest sets of muscles in your entire body… therefore they are the easiest to relax.

Beginning to count now - 1 - 2 - 3 - begin to relax the tiny muscles in and around your eyes… that's right… just let them relax deeply… feeling good.

Now... take a deep breath - and as you exhale, give your body permission to relax ten times deeper than you are right now… just let go… allowing all the tension of the day to just slip away… to slip right out of your body.

And from this moment on, you will relax completely - easily and naturally - and with each word that I say - you will go deeper and deeper relaxed.

Doing so, very, very well… so very, very calm… so very, very relaxed. So very, very comfortable… so very… very… peaceful that it's all so calm, and oh so… peaceful… we are really at peace now… you're at peace with yourself… and feeling wonderful.

I would like you now to imagine a large cloud… a large fluffy white cloud - this is the cloud of forgetfulness - this cloud is made just for you… it's for you… to put in all of those things that you would just as soon let go of… things that no longer serve you… like excess baggage.

You have carried it around with you for a very, very long time… it's time to let it go… set it down… all those worries and troubles… it's time to let go.

And from this moment on you feel more peaçeful… more tranquil… take a moment and place all of the things into the cloud that you find you no longer need… take a moment…

Pause

And as soon as you realize you've placed all that you feel like placing into your cloud - all that no longer serves you… then just watch as the cloud drifts away… watch as it floats up into the sky… taking all your cares and worries with it… watching as it rises higher and higher.

See yourself now and in the future… doing all of the things you want to do and become the person you want to be, can be and will be the person you deserve to be.

Understand that the triple warmer meridian is unique in that it is not energetically tied to a specific organ in the body ... In fact, this meridian helps to regulate all the organs and energy in the body ... this is why the triple warmer is often referred to as the organ with function, but no form....

Allow yourself to see that your key to achieving your dreams and desires lies in your understanding that you are the keeper of your joy and happiness, the key to knowing yourself and what you want and why, which in turn has the capacity to deliver the best you…

Become aware of the fact that you cannot control the outer world, understand that control of the outer world is an illusion ... and better understanding your meridians positions you to gain far greater control of your inner world…

Know that the triple warmer is the official in charge of irrigation, metabolic passage of water, Yuan, or original, Qi and prenatal Qi ... water makes up about 70 percent of the human body, so the distribution of this water is very important to the smooth operation of human life ... the triple warmer governs all the Qi of internal organs and meridians: inside and outside, left and right, and upper and lower...

Bring your awareness to the fact that for over the course of 2,500 years, Traditional Chinese Medicine has become a tried and tested system of rational medicine known for its great diversity of healing and wellness practices ... know that the main goal of TCM is to create harmony between our mind, body, and the environment around us ...

Understand that one very important way to create harmony is by making sure your Qi is balanced ... Qi means life energy and it stands for the energy in all things...

Your Qi provides the energy for important bodily functions like your digestion, metabolism, and overall strength ... It is also represented in other physical aspects of energy like your phone, sunlight, and electricity ... But other aspects like your thoughts and emotions are also powered by your Qi....

Let your mind drift to the magic of the meridians and how they work like a network system, transporting and distributing Qi and blood ... how the meridians link up organs, limbs, joints, bones, tendons, tissues and skin, and provide communication between the body interior and exterior, through a healthy meridian system...

Marvel at the magic of how Qi and blood successfully warm and nourish different organs and tissues, and maintain normal metabolic activities...

Understand that meridians are essential in supporting the flow of nutritive Qi inside the blood vessels and flow of protective Qi around them ... they strengthen the body's immunity, protect against external pernicious influences and assist in regulating Yin and Yang ...

Your Qi can become unbalanced due to a lack of nutritious food, clean, mineralized water, good sleep, and fresh air ... By nourishing your body and staying in harmony with your environment, you'll be able to restore and balance your Qi ... nutritious food... restorative sleep... herbal teas... time spent in nature... and of course meditation can all serve to balance your

Qi… and so can deep breathing and of course acupuncture… be kind to yourself… engage in activities that that serve to balance your Qi…

Give yourself permission to embrace a new awareness of your power to create reality through the balancing your Qi and your meridians through meditation and how this awareness will prepare you to live unconditionally…

Notice the happiness you feel inside knowing how powerful meridian balance is and how connected to humanity you are…notice how this connection fills you with an elevated vibration… and how an elevated vibration can expand the visible spectrums of your senses…

Now just breathe and be with yourself and let the waves of your breathing be with you…

CHAPTER ELEVEN

Gallbladder Meridian

Characteristics

The gallbladder is the organ responsible for decision making and is similar to an official of justice and integrity, an official that takes decisions.

The power of the gallbladder is integrity, discernment, daring and decisive.

From eleven pm to one am, meridian Qi mainly flows through the gall bladder meridian. This is the best time to sleep.

Regenerate.

If you have a gallstone, you'll likely become aware of it during this time!

The Ancient Chinese called the gallbladder meridian the "Honorable Minister."

While the liver plans, the gall bladder decides and discerns.

People rely on courage to seek good luck and avoid negative evil energy. Only by keeping upright can one seek good luck and avoid evil. The benevolent must be courageous, and the courage comes from the gallbladder.

When the gallbladder is strong then people's actions are bold and correct. If gallbladder Qi is weak, although thinking a lot with good deliberation, but unable to make decisions, things are ultimately difficult to achieve.

There are few important concepts regarding the gallbladder meridian in TCM.

Gallbladder meridian flows from the head to the side of the body like a door hinge. It is the hub for lifting and exiting of the human body's Qi machine. It can adjust the function of the viscera and Qi, which is very important in the twelve-meridian system.

If the gallbladder meridian is in an unfavorable state a variety of problems can arise such as migraine, ribs pain, hip and back pain.

Eleven pm to one am is the gallbladder meridian time. At this time, it's like seeds are just sprouting, all the organs' transportation and growth must rely on the gallbladder's power generated. If you do not sleep, you will feel very tired the next day, and even if you sleep more during the day, it will not be returned, because the organ's function has been damaged. In the long run, you will suffer from many diseases, and the health care must understand this truth.

The gallbladder and the heart are connected.

The heart is responsible for spirit and mental activity; the gallbladder is responsible for decisiveness. Ambition is held in the gallbladder. In the mind, both complement each other and use each other.

Clinically, if gallbladder is sick, the gallbladder Qi will raise up to disturb the heart. Palpitations, fearfulness, sleepiness or sleeplessness.

As a result, clinically, heart palpitation can treat gallbladder.

Viscera depends on the gallbladder and the human body is like a car in that the gallbladder is equivalent to the ignition, the heart is like the engine, the kidney is like the fuel trunk. The gallbladder decision starts a new journey. But where should we go? It all depends on gallbladder's upright decision. If not, we will go down the evil road and face new dangers, this is the meaning of the gallbladder upright decision, starting life and guiding life in the right way.

If there is sickness there is a reason we have ignored: we are not upright, without integrity.

Not only can it cause gallbladder problems it can cause all diseases. Are we being honest with ourselves? Are we being honest with others? Are we handling stress? Do we not live up to our potential because we fear power?

We can fall out of integrity through selfishness and timidity.

Many times, we dare not tell the truth; it was only the little boy who dared to say that the emperor did not wear clothes, and adults cheered.

This is the truth of life. It is also the root of our disease. It is to punish our hypocrisy and selfishness. To punish yourself you become a "yes" man. We don't dare to face life; life lets us feel pain and regret.

Some people say: if one faces life head on will they not die? Yes, they will not only die, they will die even earlier, but they will not be tortured to death by evil diseases.

Because they died heroically, their Qi was magnificent, and blood was warm. Just because such a person exists, we will honor the heroes, respect justice, and respect them so that we know that people can have a worthwhile life.

Gallbladder engages in storage of biliary, a fine, clean, bitter, yellow-green brush. Bile is related to the digestive absorption function of the small intestine and participates in digestion. However, gallbladder does not participate in digestion, does not deal with waste, food, drink or transport nourishment.

The gallbladder secretes bile to aid in digestion for muscular energy and works with the lymphatic system to clear out lactic acid. It follows that the gallbladder meridian is in part responsible for muscular health.

Gall bladder Meridian

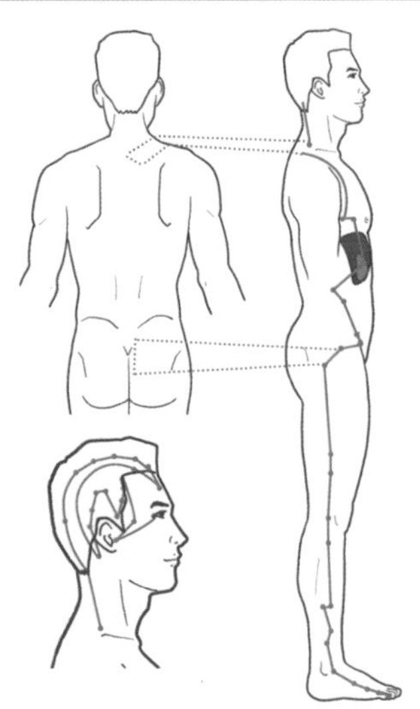

Primary Pathway

The gallbladder meridian starts from the outer corner of the eye and divides into two branches. One branch runs externally and weaves back and forth at the lateral side of the head, goes inside of the ear, then comes out the front of the ear, After curving behind the ear, it reaches the top of the shoulder and crosses the lateral side of the rib cage and abdomen, until it ends up at the side of the hip.

The other branch enters the cheek and runs internally downward, through the neck and chest to connect with the gallbladder. It continues moving downwards and comes out in the lower abdomen, where it connects with the other branch at the hip.

The hip branch then runs toward the lateral side of the thigh and lower leg. After crossing the ankle, it goes over the foot to reach the tip of the fourth toe.

Another small branch leaves the meridian and terminates at the big toe to connect with the liver meridian.

The gallbladder meridian starts from the outer corner of the eye... People with protruding temples are stubborn. The meridians must be symmetrical, so as long as there are asymmetrical spots and pains on the body, it is a meridian disease.

Main Indications

Acupuncture points in this meridian are indicated for ailments of the eyes, ears, pharynx (throat), and lateral side of the head in addition to mental illness and fever. They are also recommended for symptoms along the meridian's pathway.

An imbalance in the gallbladder meridian generates more mental afflictions than physical. Such an imbalance leads to insomnia and stiffness of the muscles. It can also cause poor judgment, timidity, and indecision.

Symptoms

In TCM, the gallbladder is closely related to the liver. Hence, the disharmony of the gallbladder meridian causes symptoms such as:

Bitter taste in the mouth.

Sigh. A sigh is caused by the upward reversal of the bile, and the gallbladder meridian travels through the diaphragm, so once the gallbladder Qi is insufficient and cannot rise, people like to sigh or let out a long sigh of relief.

Rib pain. When someone cannot be turned to the side, or cannot turn when they lie in bed. This is the manifestation of heart problems on the gallbladder meridian.

The face looks very dirty, not clean. Body skin is not moisturized. In fact, the Yang Qi of the gallbladder cannot be produced, and it cannot be distributed to the whole body.

Malaria. Malaria is cold and hot alternated, Chinese medicine classic formula Xiao Chai Hu herb tea can help.

Lymphadenopathy and cervical lymphadenitis. These diseases that are mostly on the side of the human body travel along the gallbladder meridian and must be treated from the gallbladder.

Headache and pain at the outer angle of the eyelids, jaw pain. Because the gallbladder meridian originates from the sharp canthus of the eye, the upper corner of the head, and the lower cheek.

Gallbladder governs bone disease. All bone problems need to be addressed through the gallbladder meridian. That is, as long as there is a problem with the bones in the body, it must be looked at from the perspective of gallbladder disease. The kidney also dominates the bones. In fact, the bone has bone and marrow. Whether the bone is hard or not depends on the kidney essence. Whether the bone marrow can grow or not depends on the gallbladder.

Gallbladder meridian enters the hip joint, the femoral head, and the flank ribs. These places are all bones. Therefore, if there are bone diseases, bone metastases, etc., we must pay attention to the gallbladder.

Pain along the meridian pathway such as in the axilla (armpit), chest, lower chest, buttocks and the lateral side of the lower limbs can also indicate a disorder of the gallbladder meridian. As long as the large joints in our body hurt, it is a gallbladder problem. Look at our big joints: two wrists, two elbows, two shoulders, two hips, two knees, and two ankles. These twelve joints correspond to the 12 months. When massaging or stretching, we should loosen these 12 big joints first, so that the whole body can be healed.

If you can't fall asleep or are angry, circle your ankles and wrists first, and it will relieve tension in the upper body and empty the mind to help you fall asleep. Aging starts from the legs and feet, therefore, you have to turn your ankles, your knees, and your hips so that the Yang Qi can move. That's why stretching, yoga and tai chi are more important lifestyles than body work out as we get older. If a child has poor concentration, turning his ankles every day can also calm his Qi.

Dizziness. When the gallbladder Yang Qi cannot be generated the blood supply to the brain will be insufficient because the gallbladder must be used to bring the liver blood to the head.

Gallbladder is like an igniter. Viscera depends on gallbladder Qi growth, but who is the one to activate this igniter? It relies on *Spirit*. The real owner of the car is the person, not the car. Only when the human spirit is sufficient the Yang energy can be activated and the car can be driven on the correct track. When people get old, they lack Shen and spirits are timid, and the car becomes unstable.

Since *Spirits* are the masters of the body, let's talk about the ***five spirits in TCM***.

That is:

The heart spirit is spirit (Shen)

The liver spirit is the soul, (Hun)

The lung Spirit is the soul, (Po)

The spleen Spirit is the mind (Yi)

The kidney Spirit is the will (Zhi)

Heart stores mind (Shen), Lung stores corporeal soul (Po), Liver stores ethereal soul (Hun), Spleen stores thought (Yi), Kidney stores will power (Zhi). These are so called the five storages.

Let's talk about the soul first. In Chinese, Soul has Hun and Po, there are no equivalent words to it in English.

Hun is Yang energy, which constitutes human thinking and intelligence.

Po is the rough and turbid Yin that constitutes the human body.

The twelve meridians originate from the Lung Meridian and end in the Liver Meridian.

The Lung spirit is the soul (Hun). If the soul (Hun) is insufficient, a person cannot be born.

The liver spirit is the soul (Po). Liver spirit (Po) stays, the person won't die. The so-called "boldness" refers to the power of human instinct, courage is innate, and ability is cultivated in life. A person with ability is not necessarily courageous.

Usually, when we describe a person's mental outlook or ability, we often say: This person has courage, this person has willpower, etc. What do these mean?

Remember, Chinese medicine looks at people, and there are *essence* aspects, such as physical strength and physical endurance. There is also the level of Qi such as high-spiritedness, ease and calmness, etc. There is also a *spirit* level, such as calmness, extraordinary concentration, and great wisdom.

What does human achievement have to do with it? Now the argument is related to human intelligence and emotional intelligence. Let's look at this question from the perspective of TCM. It must be related to *spirit*, *Qi*, and *essence*". If there is only essence, but no spirit and no Qi, it is a reckless man. Only when the spirit, Qi, and essence are all strong, can one have a rich imagination, strong memory, extraordinary willpower, and concentration. Only in this way can we achieve success and connect to higher wisdom.

When a person is full of energy and spirit, he has the power and energy to think; when the liver and gallbladder are strong, his imagination and creativity are strong; when the spleen is full, the relevance and his thinking is rich; the kidney is responsible for storage and collection. When kidney spirit is sufficient, a person has concentration and is grounded.

The spleen spirit is mind, and the mind has a memory and the process of further forming desire is called mind. Anyone with a strong spleen will have a rich imagination, and can make things to the extreme of an artist. An artist's imagination can be a time-space combination of completely unrelated things, while ordinary people's imagination has to have cause and effect. This is the difference between artists and everyone else. The reason why artists' artworks are expensive is because of creativity. And nonartist thoughts are generally just a continuation of cause and effect, not much creativity.

What is "zhi"? "The existence of the will is called the *zhi*, that is, the process in which the desire has been preserved and determined to be implemented, which is called the will.

Mind and will are a bit like the relationship between the spleen and the kidney. The ability to settle down and store the will is called zhi, and the kidney will be the secret treasure. The so-called willpower is to be able to relate and persist. If there is a strong connection, there will be strong creativity. If you have the willpower, you can execute and do it, and you can succeed.

Being smart means seeing a lot and listening a lot. There are not many fools in the world, but seeing a lot and listening a lot is useless if you don't have your own basic willpower. Without willpower you won't be successful. So when we understand this, we should understand that cultivating a child's willpower is much more important than cultivating them to learn well. Being smart and learning well is just an ordinary ability, but firm willpower is the ability to succeed.

Therefore, willpower is the persistence of one's own Qi and blood. Being able to persist in doing one thing is called willpower. For example, we held weekly online mediation classes for more than two years with our willpower. We did this because we believed that many people could benefit. We were not only just the hosts, at the same time, we were also looking for improvement, too. That is how success comes. Persistence and resilience, as well as execution, and the ability to put ideas into practice. This is called willpower.

Therefore, the difference between people is in their divinity. Human nature has something in common, and they all have some selfishness, greed, and attachment, but divinity determines how much you can get rid of these undesirable traits of selfishness, greed and attachment.

The so-called cultivation is to cultivate the five spirits, that is, to cultivate the greatness and breadth of our "divine nature."

When the gallbladder is strong then people's actions are bold and correct. If gallbladder Qi is weak, although thinking a lot with good deliberation, but unable to make decisions, things are ultimately difficult to achieve. Gallbladder meridian balance depends on and asks us to cultivate the five spirits. In so doing we strengthen gallbladder Qi and cultivate the greatness and breadth of "divine nature."

Gallbladder is considered an Extraordinary Organ. B

Before we explain Extraordinary Organ, let's understand the TCM Viscera called ***"Zang Fu" system*** first.

The Zang-Fu is a collection of organs that produce and regulate Qi within the body. Unlike in Western medicine, these organs should not be thought of as anatomical structures, but rather as interconnected functions that explain how Qi is produced within the body. The functions performed by each organ are referred to as the organ's Qi. In total, there are 11 organs, five Zang and six Fu, and 6 Extraordinary Organs.

Zang organs: Zang refers to the five organs that are Yin. Collectively, their primary purpose is to produce and store Qi, blood, body fluids, essence, and spirit. They are the: heart, spleen, lung, kidney and liver.

Fu organs: Fu refers to six organs that are Yang. Collectively, their primary function is to transmit and digest nutrients without storing them and to excrete waste. They are: stomach, small intestine, large intestine, bladder, gallbladder and triple warmer.

Six Extraordinary Organs: marrow, brain, bone, uterus, vessels and gallbladder.

These six Extraordinary Organs are born from the Qi of the earth, and they can store the Yin essence in the same way that the earth contains all things. Therefore, their function is to store but not excrete them, and they are called Extraordinary Organs.

The Extraordinary Organs are definitely different from the six Fu organs. What's the difference? First, the six Fu-organs are Yang, which is expelled but not stored. The brain, marrow, bones, veins, gallbladder, and uterus are named Fu organs. They all have the characteristic of "storing but not excretion." This means that they are a kind of relatively airtight human tissue, not in direct contact with water and food, that is, they are like Fu-organs but they are not Fu-organs; at the same time, they have the function of storing essence and Qi, similar to the five Zang organs, that is, they are like viscera but not Zang-organs, so they are considered strange and always maintain their own special state, so they are referred to as Extraordinary Organs.

Except for the gallbladder, which belongs to the six Fu-organs, none of the strange and constant Fu-organs have an external and internal relationship with the Five Zangs. However, some of them are related to the Eight-Meridian. Most of them are hollow in shape and resembling a Fu-organ, and their functions are capable of storing essence and Qi. For example, in the uterus, is the uterus empty? It is empty. Although she is empty, she is able to give birth to children and store the essence of life, so she also is solid. She always has a peculiar image that is neither pure Yin nor pure Yang, so they are called Extraordinary Organs.

Because the gallbladder does not receive food and water like other Fu organs and does not communicate with the exterior, gallbladder is the most extraordinary organ in six Fu organs.

Acupoints

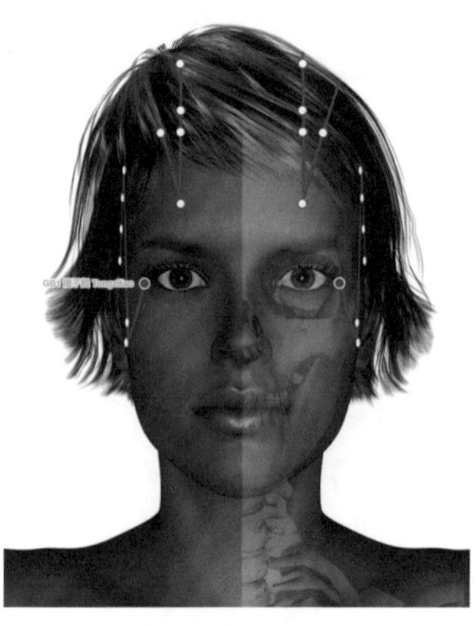

GB 1 TONG ZI LIAO (PUPIL'S BONE HOLE)

Name: Pupil's Bone Hole, Tong Zi also means child/sage that is beginning and ready to open - innocent - to see the world in a new way

Location: 0.5 cun lateral to the outer canthus of the eye, in the depression on the lateral side of the orbit.

Indication: Migraine headache around temple, side headache, red, dry, painful, burning eyes, failing of vision, loss of vision.

Technique and notes: massage

Gallbladder and triple warmer pass eye bags, gallbladder Qi strong, and triple warmer is efficient, water metabolization is efficient, there are no eye bags, having eye bags, it is insufficient Yang. The secret for the eye bags is massage GB- 1

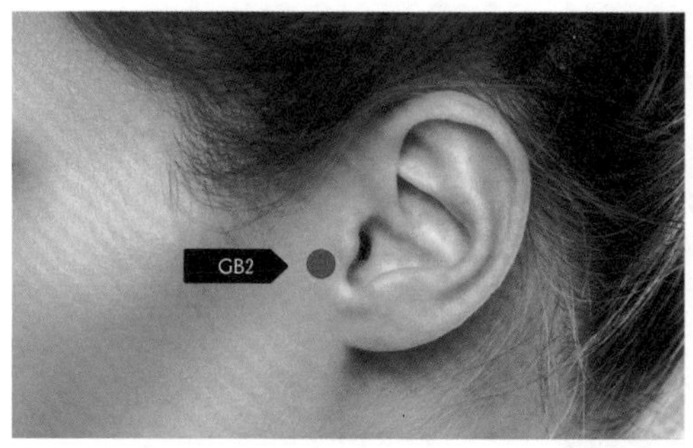

GB 2 TING HUI (AUDITORY CONVERGENCE)

Name: Auditory Convergence, do I hear what people say? Area where meridians converge into the ear

Location: Anterior to the intertragic notch of the ear, at the posterior border of the condyloid process of the mandible. The point is located with the mouth open.

Indication: tinnitus, deafness, toothache, motor impairment of TMJ, headache, etc.

Heart and gallbladder are connected. The heart is open to two ears. This heart orifice is in the ear.

The gallbladder meridian curving behind the ear, goes inside of the ear, then comes out the front of ear… The disease of the ear is closely related to the gallbladder, because gallbladder is the only meridian that goes inside the ear.

Nowadays, a large number of young people have more tinnitus, which is related to consuming a large number of cold drinks, stress and anxiety.

Ear protection exercise: insert the both middle fingers (pericardium meridian) into the ear first while finger nail facing forward, then slowly rotate until the belly of the finger is facing forward.

At this time. The finger is gently pressed inside. If there is a sticky feeling at this time, it means that the body is heavily damp. After pressing suddenly to pull it out, the ear will feel clear and relaxed right away.

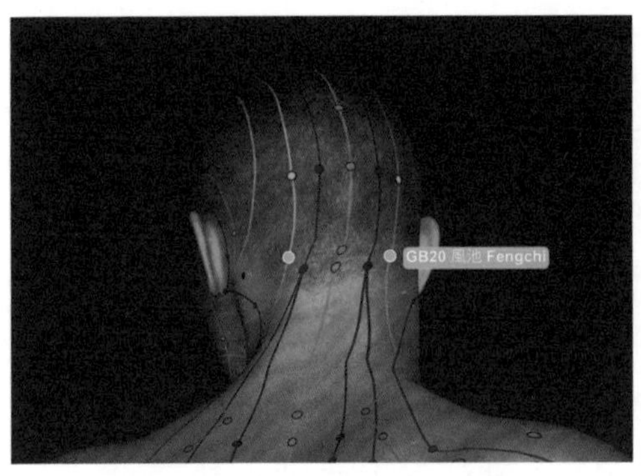

GB 20 FENG CHI (WIND POOL)

Name: Wind Pool, depression in the back of the head. The pool that collects wind. The ability to move, flow and change with a situation. Wind is movement and change.

Location: On the back of the head, in the depression between the upper portion of m. sternocleidomastoid and m. trapezius, on the same level with Du-16.

Indications: headache, dizziness, insomnia, neck pain, shoulder pain, blurred vision, glaucoma, high blood pressure, lock jaw, red or painful eyes, night blindness, tinnitus, sinus, deafness, stroke, facial nerve damage, malaria, etc.,

Technique and Notes: Massage or Jade scraper. Especially at beginning of cold, press this point, it's very sore,

This area of the neck cannot have blockage, once it is blocked, lightly can have migraine, severe can be Alzheimer. .so, it's very important to use a jade scraper to scrap this area often.

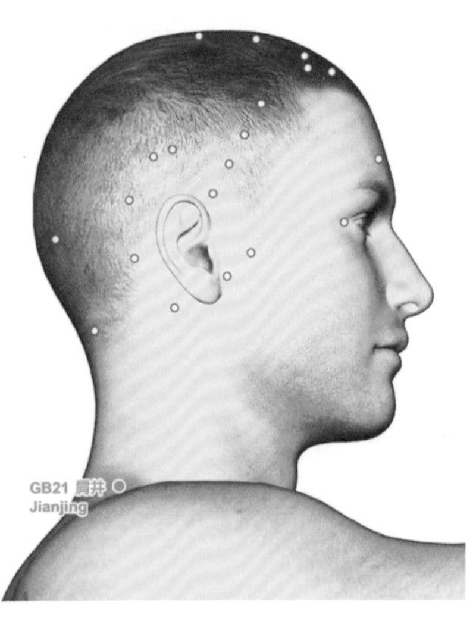

GB 21 JIAN JING (THE SHOULDER WELL)

Name: Shoulder Well: Anatomical location.

Location: AT the shoulder's highest point, same line with nipple.

Indication: Pain and rigidity in neck, pain in shoulder and back, impairment of arm attending shoulder pain, upper limbs, neck pain, etc. shoulder neck upper limb disease, and mastitis, etc. It usually is very hard here, so the starting

point of the back massage is to massage the shoulder well first.
Technique and Notes: Massage or jade scraper.

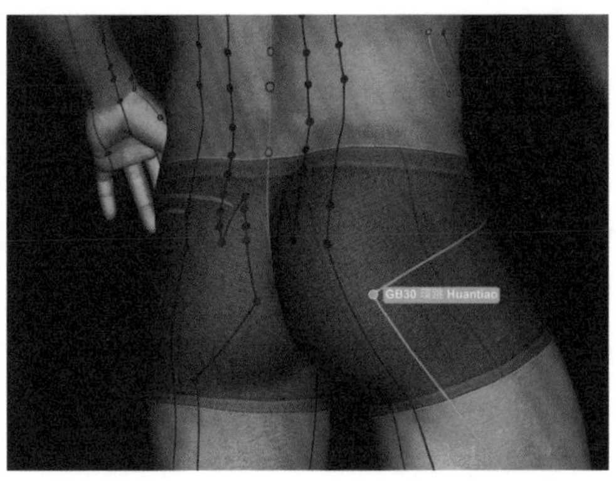

GB 30 HUAN TIAO (ENCIRCLING LEAP)

Name: Encircling Leap, easily startled, wind, Parkinson's, spasms, lock knee
Location: All the junction of the lateral one third and medial two thirds of the distance between the greater trochanter and the hiatus of the sacrum. When location the point, put the patient in recumbent position with the thigh flexed
Indication: Pain in lumbar, pain in leg, knee pain, muscular atrophy, sciatic, low energy, itchy, anus or groin, vaginal discharge, urethritis.
Technique and notes: massage or Moxibustion.

Gallbladder passed through hip. Therefore, the femoral head necrosis and any hip problems are not only related to the kidney, but also related to lack of growth of gallbladder Qi.

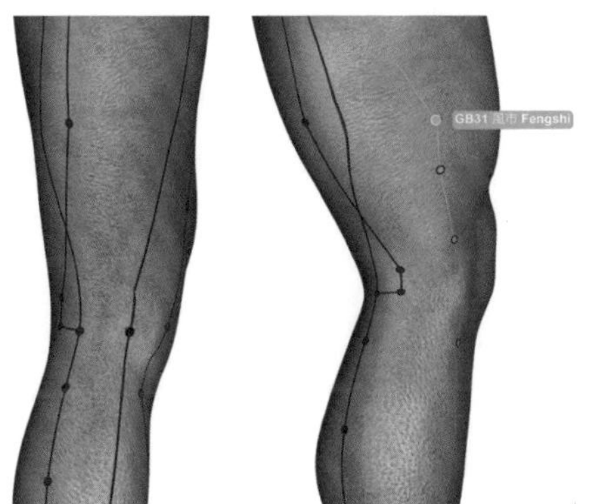

GB 31 FENG SHI (WIND'S MARKET)

Name: Wind's Market, a place where wind collects and moves. An area where change and movement can occur.
Location: On the midline of the lateral aspect of the thigh. When one is standing erect with the hand close to the sides, the point in here the tip of the middle finger rests.
Indication: Stroke, Pain and soreness in thigh and lumbar region,

paralysis of lower limbs, beriberi, rashes, moving rashes, urticaria, in the outside of the thigh, the same is at the heart of the wind, the stroke, half-length, the lower limbs, the numbness, but itchy, athlete.
Technique and notes: massage or Moxibustion, scraping.
Jade scraper to scrap this point can relieve leg pain and itching.

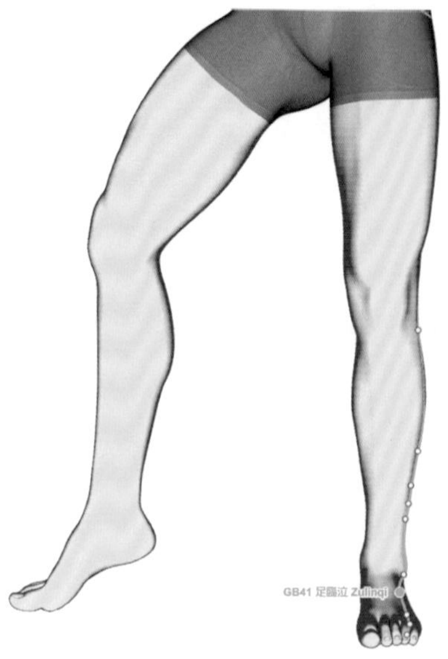

GB 41 ZU LIN XI (FOOT OVERLOOKING TEARS)

Name: Foot Overlooking Tears, it is here that the gallbladder channel breaks off and connects with the liver channel.
Location: In the depression distal to the junction of the fourth and fifth metatarsal bones, on the lateral side of the tendon of m. extensor digiti minimi of the foot.
Indication: headache, Vertigo, low back pain, muscle spasm, eye disease, cholecystitis, stroke, neurological function, breast pain, irregular menstruation, vaginal discharge etc.
Technique and notes: massage the top of our feet should not be cold, because the top of our feet are all Yang meridian, if it feels cold, that means Yang Qi are weak, some people can have charlie horse, cramps, restless legs, so foot soaking at night is very important.

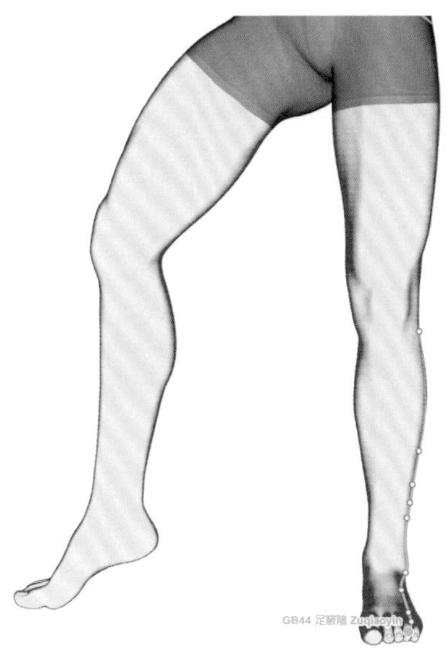

GB 44 ZU QIAO YING (FOOT PORTAL YIN)

Name: Foot Portal Yin, this is an area in the foot that helps in treating the sensory orifices.

Indication: Migraines, headache, deafness, tinnitus, dream disturbed sleep, febrile disease, insomnia, red eyes, sore throat.

Location: 0.1 cun posterior to the corner of the nail, on the lateral side of the fourth toe.

Technique and notes: massage, moxibustion.

There is another branch that enters the big toe from GB 41, it connects to the liver meridian at big toe. So, the next meridian is the liver meridian.

Ok, to summarize it, the gallbladder is the longest meridian of the body, and the meridian has 44 points on the left and right. There are a total of 88 points.

How do you take care of the gallbladder meridian?

Tapping. As we learn about the meridians, we know that the gallbladder starts at the side of the eyes, stopping at the little toe, so tapping the gallbladder to start from the side of the eyes, and gently tap both sides, don't forget to tap both sides of ribs, to waist. At the waist, grab it then release it, it can help lose weight and flatten your tummy.

Then tap all the way down the side of legs to the side of feet. After tapping, the leg will be relaxed and lighter.

Miscellaneous bits:

There are 44 points on either side for a total of 88 points.

Element: Wood
Direction: East
Season: Spring
Climate: Windy
Cultivation: Germinate
Time: 11 p.m. – 1 a.m.
Sense Organ: Eyes
Sense: Sight
Tissue: Tendons
Positive Emotion: Kindness
Negative Emotion: Anger
Flavor: Sour
Color: Yellow Green
Sound: Shouting
Smell: Scorched
Opposite: Heart
Yin/Yang: Yang
Flow Direction: Down
Origin/Ending: Face to Foot

Gallbladder Meditation

Take three slow, deep breaths and prepare yourself for a meditative journey…

Make yourself comfortable… and focus your attention onto the sound of my voice...

As you listen now, I would like you to become aware of your body and tune into your breath...

Short pause.

Now - gently close your eyes and allow yourself to become as comfortable as you possibly can.

Take another nice deep breath - and just exhale - and as you do - give yourself permission to relax.

And each time that you give yourself permission to relax - notice how your body responds - easily - quickly.

Notice how your understanding has expanded to see that the key to achieving your dreams and desires lies in your willingness to live in integrity and be decisive, the key to knowing yourself and what you want and why, which in turn has the capacity to deliver balanced Qi and health…

Become aware of the fact that you cannot control the outer world, understand that control of the outer world is an illusion...

Bring your awareness to learning that meditation, quiet stillness, is the gateway to "the zone"… know that mastering this recognition places you into the position that will allow you to create your reality; with practice, any mindstate can be tamed in meditation… any dream imagined and set in motion through the setting of intention…

Give yourself permission to dive deeply into the practice of meditation… give yourself permission to believe that if you can hold it in your mind, you can hold it in your body… to recognize where you are with your intentions and no matter where that is, you can redirect them into positive and loving thoughts for yourself and for others…

And you can feel really happy that you made the decision to come here today; taking that first important step towards understanding that balanced gallbladder meridian Qi comes from the courage of your convictions, from living your truth and that overcoming indecisiveness can lead to better overall health...

In the past, maybe you sometimes found it difficult to make decisions and stick by them, but the past is past and now you're really beginning to look forward to a wonderful future in which you're in control… a future where you honor your truth and stand in integrity…

Because you and you alone have your own best interests at heart and only you, nobody else, can possibly know exactly what you're thinking or feeling or going to do ...

And you are going to surprise yourself and others with your newly found confidence and ability to make decisions, whether large or small, in your life...

Understand that the gallbladder is the organ responsible for decision making and is similar to an official of justice and integrity, an official that makes decisions ... The power of the gallbladder is integrity, discernment, daring and decisive....

Allow yourself to see that your key to achieving your dreams and desires lies in your understanding that you are the keeper of your courage and authentic voice, the key to knowing yourself and what you want and why, which in turn has the capacity to deliver the best you…

Become aware of the fact that you cannot control the outer world, understand that control of the outer world is an illusion ... and better understanding your meridians positions you to gain far greater control of your inner world…

Know that the Ancient Chinese called the Gallbladder meridian the Honorable Minister ... while the liver plans, the gall bladder decides and discerns ... people rely on courage to seek good luck and avoid negative evil energy ... and only by keeping upright one can seek good luck and avoid evil, the benevolent must be courageous, and the courage comes from the gallbladde ...

When the gallbladder is strong then people's actions are bold and correct ... If gallbladder Qi is weak, although thinking a lot with good deliberation, but unable to make decisions, things are ultimately difficult to achieve....

Bring your awareness to the fact that for over the course of 2,500 years, Traditional Chinese Medicine has become a tried and tested system of rational medicine known for its great diversity of healing and wellness practices ... know that the main goal of TCM is to create harmony between our mind, body, and the environment around us ...

Understand that one very important way to create harmony is by making sure your Qi is balanced ... Qi means life energy and it stands for the energy in all things ...

Your Qi provides the energy for important bodily functions like your digestion, metabolism, and overall strength ... It is also represented in other physical aspects of energy like your phone, sunlight, and electricity ... But other aspects like your thoughts and emotions are also powered by your Qi....

Let your mind drift to the magic of the meridians and how they work like a network system, transporting and distributing Qi and blood ... how the meridians link up organs, limbs, joints, bones, tendons, tissues and skin, and provide communication between the body interior and exterior, through a healthy meridian system...

Marvel at the magic of how Qi and blood successfully warm and nourish different organs and tissues, and maintain normal metabolic activities...

Understand that meridians are essential in supporting the flow of nutritive Qi inside the blood vessels and flow of protective Qi around them ... they strengthen the body's immunity, protect against external pernicious influences and assist in regulating Yin and Yang ...

Your Qi can become unbalanced due to a lack of nutritious food, clean, mineralized water, good sleep, and fresh air ... By nourishing your body and staying in harmony with your environment, you'll be able to restore and balance your Qi ... nutritious food... restorative sleep... herbal teas... time spent in nature... and of course meditation can all serve to balance your Qi... and so can deep breathing and of course acupuncture... be kind to yourself... engage in activities that that serve to balance your Qi...

Give yourself permission to embrace a new awareness of your power to create reality through the balancing your Qi and your meridians through meditation and how this awareness will prepare you to live unconditionally...

Understand that not only can being indecisive or living out of integrity cause gallbladder problems it can cause all diseases ... ask yourself routinely if you are being honest with yourself... if you are being honest with others… are you handling stress… are you not living up to your potential because you fear power… we can fall out of integrity through selfishness and timidity ... understand how important courage to be yourself, to stand up for yourself and to speak your truth is to the health of your gallbladder meridian and to health generally…

Know that the gallbladder is like an igniter ... but who activates this igniter? It relies on Spirit… Only when the human spirit is sufficient the yang energy can be activated and the car can be driven on the correct track...

Notice the happiness you feel inside knowing how powerful meridian balance is and how connected to humanity you are…notice how this connection fills you with an elevated vibration… and how an elevated vibration can expand the visible spectrums of your senses…

Now just breathe and be with yourself and let the waves of your breathing be with you…

CHAPTER TWELVE

Liver Meridian

Characteristics

The liver is considered one of the primary organs in TCM. It is called the "Chief of Staff" and official of the General.

The liver is an important organ responsible for the metabolism of the human body to keep the human body youthful, energetic and healthy.

In TCM, the liver has a complex interaction with the other organs and this meridian and its impact leads TCM to approach the liver with a holistic view and to see it as the liver system.

From one am to three am, meridian Qi mainly flows through the Liver meridian. This is a time for deep rest and dreaming.

If you wake up at this time your liver is overwhelmed by detoxifying.

Alcohol, chemicals, drugs, poor diet all call on the liver to detox!

In Western medicine, the liver is an organ with metabolic functions and it plays a full role in detoxification, storage of glycogen, synthesis of secretory proteins, etc. The liver is an important organ responsible for the metabolism of the human body to keep the human body youthful, energetic and healthy.

The liver in TCM medical theory includes not only the liver organ as in Western medicine, but also the liver meridian, liver Qi, the relationship between other organs, as well as the interaction between the liver and the gallbladder, heart fire, etc.

These are collectively called the "liver system," which is part of a bigger, holistic view. From this point of view, it is far more complex than Western medicine perception of the liver.

The liver is the officer of the general and the mastermind.

That is to say, the liver is like a general, strategizing. It must have intelligence. It depends on a strong essence and growth energy. Only having essence is not enough, it will still be sluggish.

Therefore, among the five Zang- organs, the liver has the most growth energy. In life, liver the general, arranges for vitality.

A person's discomfort stems from the suffocation of the liver. Anger and depression cause suffocation of the liver's vitality. The ultimate loss of vitality is when a person dies, which means that there is no vitality at all.

Of the five elements the liver belongs to wood. The nature of wood is straight, that is to say, the power of growth is straight, and the power of convergence is curved. The balance of these two abilities is called wood. If there is only growth, without the convergence, it will cause a disease of the body, that is, hyperactivity of liver Yang. People who have excessive growth will become dizzy, because only when they come up, without the essence to moisten the head, there will be more dandruff, the scalp will be itchy, and the hair will fall out.

When many people are anxious, they suppress the growth of essence. As a result, sleep becomes a problem, and lack of sleep affects immunity the most. Follow nature, go to bed when it is dark, get up at sunrise, not against the natural flow, and don't let yourself get too tired.

Exhaustion damages the liver, excessive sexual life and overwork will hurt liver. In fact, all "tiredness" is a tired heart and resentment, its root of liver disease.

Liver and gallbladder are symbiotic. Liver is benevolence, gallbladder restrains liver's benevolence, without gallbladder's upright posture, the courage of the gallbladder will become evil; the benevolence of the liver will become unprincipled, the benevolence of the liver needs the protection of the integration with the gallbladder.

The liver stores blood. When a person lies down, the blood goes to the liver. You stand, talk, exercise, etc., all dissipates blood. Just lying down is useless. You have to close your eyes and nourish your liver. Roll the tongue to nourish the heart. Now there are many people with dry eyes and dry mouths. If you lie still for a while, your mouth will be full of saliva. At this time, if you want to get rid of all kinds of distracting thoughts, you can count your breath 36 times. When a person is asleep, the blood of the human body can be attributed to the liver and complete the metabolism.

If you close your eyes and don't fall asleep, people are still thinking about things. As long as they think about things, the liver blood has to be adjusted upwards, so we must sleep.

It's not only sleeping, but also having no dreams. The ancients said that "sages have no dreams." The so-called saints have no dreams. So you can see how difficult it is to maintain this liver blood.

When a person is lying down, blood belongs to the liver, which means that once a person falls asleep, the body's Qi and blood begin to concentrate its energy and metabolize.

When liver blood is sufficient, people's vision is good, and the eyes are bright. The feet are nourished by liver blood and can walk.

When the palm is nourished by liver blood, there is grip strength. For the elderly over 70 years old, the greater the grip strength, the longer the life. When the fingers are nourished by liver blood, they can ingest things flexibly.

Therefore, the morning stiffness of the elderly and the inability to flex and extend the fingers are all related to the lack of liver blood.

Nowadays, many people use mobile phones every day, and their finger joints are stagnant, all kinds of numbness, and stiffness.

What to do?

Put down the phone.

Every morning and evening, clench your fist 49 times. Open, clench the fist, repeat.

Moxibustion on fingers and wrists. Ten minutes a day. At the same time moxibustion Zhongwan Guanyuan. In short, let your hands serve you for a while!

Always close your eyes and rest your mind.

More sun exposure and more walking. Half an hour a day.

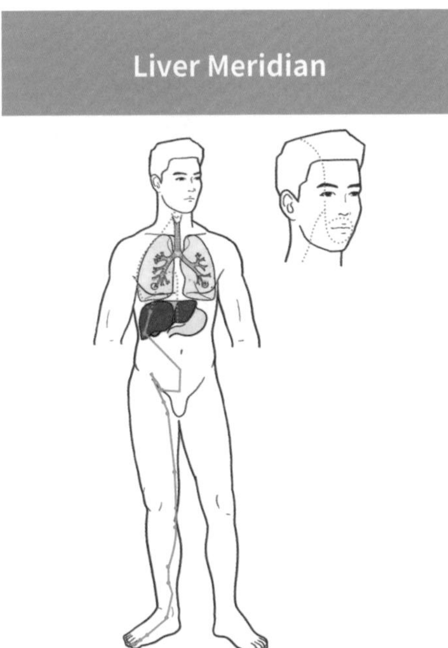

Primary Pathway

The liver meridian starts from the top of the big toe and goes across the top of the foot. After crossing the inner ankle, it continues to go upwards along the inner side of the lower leg and the thigh, until it reaches the pubic region. It then circulates around the external genitalia and enters the lower abdomen. Afterwards, it goes up the abdomen and reaches the lower chest to connect with the liver and gallbladder. The meridian further travels upwards along the throat and connects with the eyes. Finally it emerges from the forehead to reach the vertex of the head. One of its internal branches originates internally from the eye and moves downwards to the cheek where it curves around the inner surface of the lips. Another branch starts from the liver and passes through the diaphragm to reach the lung where it connects with the lung meridian and completes the cycle of the twelve meridians.

The liver meridian, in terms of the order of the twelve meridians, ranks last, but it is definitely a very important meridian among the twelve meridians, because it is related to life and death. When a person is born, he acquires the essence of the liver, so he will hold on to it and live; when a person dies, his soul will fly away, and he will let go, which is also a matter of the liver.

Main Indications

Acupuncture points in this meridian are indicated for liver, gynecological and genital diseases. They are also recommended for symptoms along the meridian's pathway.

The liver meridian is in charge of the peripheral nervous system as well as the ligaments and tendons. Hypertension and the inability to relax are caused by an imbalance in the liver meridian. Liver imbalances are diagnosed by examining the eyes or fingernails and toenails. Imbalance of this meridian can also cause anger issues.

Symptoms

Disharmony of the liver meridian leads to:

Hernias- The most common is small intestinal hernia. It is a common and frequently-occurring disease. In the treatment of hernia, we can start from the liver meridian and the Ren meridian. The cause is the depression of the liver, spleen and stomach Qi.

Both ribs are full, chest fullness, stomach and lower abdomen bloating. The liver meridian runs through the diaphragm and ribs.

Prostate: There are generally four reasons for prostate problems:

One is to retain the sperm. If a man withholds ejaculation, it is easy to cause the prostate to become enlarged. After a long time, it will become inflamed. If you encounter depression and abnormally cold energy cancer can form.

Second is being sedentary without exercising.

Also, as one ages, Yang Qi is deficient, cannot transform your essence, and one will get sick if your Qi and essence are stagnated.

Finally, today's boys have sex too early, which will damage their essence, so some people have prostate problems at a young age, and the more disordered they are, the worse they may be.

Groin pain, the lower back pain, urinary incontinence, difficulty urinating,

Anger, irritability, bad temper. Liver's negative emotion.

Sudden blindness and deafness from big anger. So it's really stupid to be angry, it's just hurting yourself. The so-called practice is really to first cultivate emotional stability, and then cultivate to maintain emotional cleanliness and stability.

Easily fearful, people with insufficient liver essence tend to become fearful, conversely people with sufficient liver essence are bold.

Dry throat is one of the characteristics of liver disease, the liver meridian goes through the throat, as has been noted.

Thyroid disease, the thyroid is an important organ for maintaining metabolism and respiratory rate. Furthermore, the neck, with the head on the top, represents rationality, and the body on the bottom, representing instinct. The long-term conflict between rationality and instinct, reality and ideal, will cause entanglement and lesions in the neck and throat. People with this kind of disease generally have high IQ, low EQ (emotional intelligence), and live too tangled. In short, this is the result of people competing with themselves or with others.

Facial dust decolorization. Liver blood deficiency can cause anemia, people can have pale complexions. The gallbladder meridian is "face like dust," cannot be washed clean, gray and not bright. The heart disease is white, that is, white and a layer of floating light. A person with a pale face will soon have a heart attack. As mentioned earlier, it is particularly important that people's face colors are not afraid of the dark, white, yellow, or red, but there must be a soft glow, like a layer of gauze.

A good complexion and good skin must have a soft glow, and this light must be restrained and not smoothed out. If it is white, it will smooth the light outside. It's a bit like matte finish and gloss finish, the gloss is all out and the matte is inward.

Liver color is blue, blue is related to fright and pain, and dark is related to lack of essence and failure of essence. It must be clearly distinguished, these two are very different. For example, if a child has blue veins on the bridge of the nose, it may be frightened in the womb. For example, when a pregnant woman steps on the air, she is shocked.

However, the exposure of blue veins near the temples of some adults is a typical liver blood deficiency.

Nourishing the liver focuses on warming the liver, and the liver controls the flow of fluids. Once medicine is taken indiscriminately, it will aggravate the metabolism of the liver and cause liver cold. So the first step for everyone to learn is to be careful when taking medication because once you take the wrong medicine, the consequences can be very serious.

There are four main reasons for liver disease:

First is a lack of vitality. Second, long-term depression and anger. In fact, all serious illnesses are emotional illnesses. Third, eating disorder. Poor diet weakens the digestion function resulting in disharmony between the liver, gallbladder, spleen and stomach. Once the vitality is insufficient, it is easy to be infected with the bacteria or virus. Finally, overwork, long term tiredness, fatigue, exhaustion, can damage the liver.

As far as the transmission law of hepatitis B is concerned, it will generally change to liver cirrhosis, liver ascites, and even liver cancer. All in all, liver disease gradually deteriorates with the gradual weakening of vitality. The principle of treatment should be to restore the function of the spleen and kidney, because the accumulation of vitality comes from a healthy spleen and stomach function and a healthy diet. At the same time, "water can generate wood," and the recovery of liver wood must rely on sufficient kidney water.

There are three reasons for the formation of fatty liver:

First, the function of the spleen Yang is weakened, and the function of the pancreas cannot function normally. Second, the high-calorie diet intake of obese patients is also a factor in the formation of fatty liver. The accumulation of fat in the liver is proportional to the body weight. After the weight control of obese patients, the degree of fatty liver will be reduced. Third, excessive drinking damages the liver.

Liver cancer: women generally don't have liver cancer. If a woman has liver cancer, she must have experienced great suffering and resentment in her life.

Men are more likely to get liver cancer than women. The reason is very simple, because the poison in the liver of women can be excreted through menstruation, while the anger and poison of men have no outlet, so men are more likely to develop liver cancer.

Acupoints

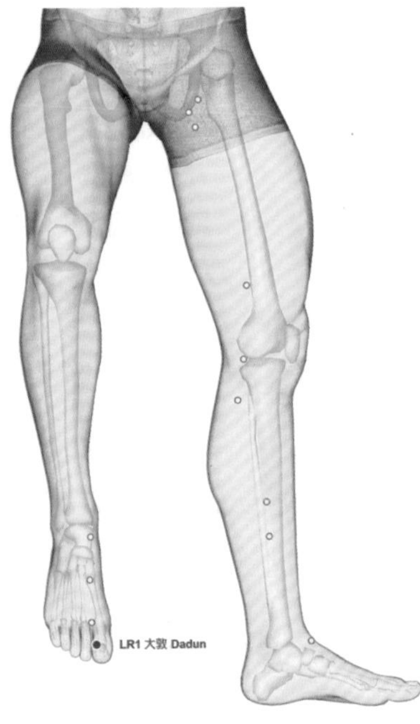

LIVER 1: DADUN (GREAT PILE)

Name: Great Pile: Clears things we have piled up especially damp heat in the lower Jiao (uterus, UTI). To let go of things that no longer serve you. As this is the last channel in the sequence, there is a severe deficiency. Therefore in order to use this point let go, use it in combination with the presenting deficiency.

Location: On the lateral side of the terminal of the big toe, between the interphalangeal joint and the lateral corner of the nail.

Indication: hernia, prolapse uterus, incontinence, Alzheimer's, menstruation problem, spotting, epilepsy, enuresis, uterine bleeding, sweating and bleeding, bed wetting, infertility, seminal loss.

Technique and notes: Massage or bleeding.

Now so many people are anxious, adults and children have trouble falling asleep, wake up in the middle of night and cannot fall back to sleep, wake up in the morning, confused, unhappy, and physically and mentally fatigued.

Acupressure applied to Dadun can make the mind clear, eyes bright, and quick-acting. During acupressure, press the Dadun point for 7-8 seconds, then slowly exhale, especially do it in the morning, about 10 times.

But all diseases of the reproductive system must be treated from the liver meridian.

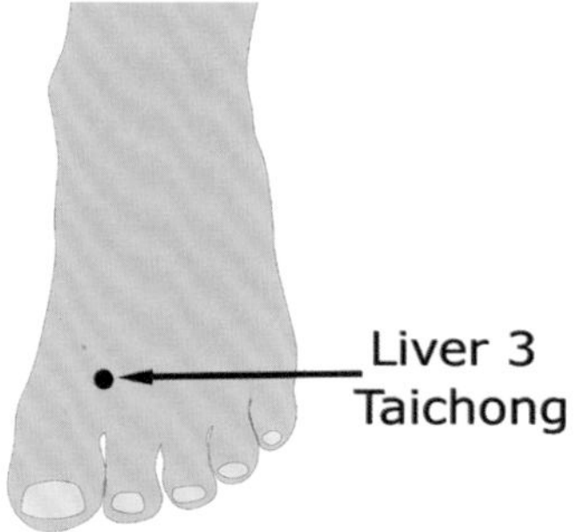

LIVER 3 TAI CHONG (GREAT SURGING)

Name: Great Surging, source point, to be able to surge and move forward. Movement in Chong Vessel, blood movement, high blood pressure, varicosity, sweating (moving fluids), sweating after birth.

Location: On the dorsum of the foot, in the depression distal to the junction of the first and second metatarsal toes, 1.5 to 2 cun above the web.

Indication: Qi stagnation, dampness, fullness, deviated mouth, red eyes, burning, itching, headache, hyperthyroid, epilepsy, eye dry, menstruation problems, uterine bleeding, hernia, headache, dizziness, vertigo, insomnia, red face, depression,

Technique and notes: Massage

Massaging the liver meridian and inner thighs also has many benefits. Except for standing, splitting and sex, we seldom touch to the inner thighs. If you massage it often, because it belongs to Yin, and the outside of the leg is Yang, the Yang things move easily, while the Yin does not move, and the Yin is easy to condense, so it is necessary to consciously massage the inner thigh.

When the liver has problems, its air flow is in the two armpits, so it is necessary to spread the two armpits.

The specific method is: cross the two palms, hold at the back of the head, and keep the hands flush with the shoulders, as far as possible to stretch and pull both arms.

This action suddenly opened the two armpits. Then, maintain this action and slowly turn left.

During the process of turning left, do not close the two armpits, turn left slowly, and hold your breath for a while when you turn to the farthest side.

Then, slowly come over and turn right again, trying desperately to look back. The eyes are also dominated by the liver, so look back.

Do it six times each day. This is a great way to relieve liver stasis.

Miscellaneous bits:

There are 14 points.
Element: Wood
Direction: East
Season: Spring
Climate: Windy
Cultivation: Germinate
Time: 1 a.m. – 3 a.m.
Sense Organ: Eyes
Sense: Sight
Tissue: Tendons
Positive Emotion: Kindness
Negative Emotion: Anger
Flavor: Sour
Color: Deep Green
Sound: Shouting
Smell: Scorched
Opposite: Small Intestine
Yin/Yang: Yin
Origin/Ending: Foot to Face
Number of points: 14 on one side of the body, total 28

Liver Meditation

Take three slow, deep breaths and prepare yourself for a meditative journey…

Make yourself comfortable… and focus your attention onto the sound of my voice...

As you listen now, I would like you to become aware of your body and tune into your breath...

Short pause.

Now, tilt your head ever so slightly to elongate your spine and open the energy system that runs through it… And now close your eyes if you haven't already done so and begin to deepen your breath…

And breathe, inhale and exhale…

Use the sound of your breath to ground you in this present moment… this here and now… And notice when you feel yourself getting lighter in your body and continue breathing… inhale and exhale… breathing in relaxation, exhaling any tension or stress…

Let go of any thoughts that come… don't fight them ... just notice them and use an exhalation to let them go… And then bring your attention back to your breath…

And back to the sound of my voice… to ground you, here and now… there is no place but here, there is no time but now… and right here and right now, I want you to inhale deeply through your nose and as you do, notice how your body expands with your breath… how your belly and chest fill up with new air…

And as you exhale, notice how your body contracts… as it releases the air and releases the tension… notice how your belly and chest fall back down and notice any sensation of release that each exhalation brings… let go of any tension or holding in the body… let it relax fully and sink into the surface beneath it… let it feel powerful… let it feel transformational…

In this moment, this here and now, you are powerful and you can transform yourself…

Allow yourself to become so relaxed and comfortable now that you can imagine or visualize yourself walking in your favorite place.

I want you to concentrate now on your breathing.

And breathe deeply and evenly, slowly and regularly.

Inhale the air deep into your lungs and hold each breath for the mental count of three.

As you do this, I want you to breathe in whatever it is that you need; whether this be hope or optimism, determination, persistence, or confidence or anything else.

And whatever it is that has been holding you back – breathe it out.

Let it go.

That's right, just let it go.

Inhale deeply in this way, three or four times, always remembering to breathe away any negativity that has been stopping you from fulfilling your dreams and accessing your vitality.

Short Pause.

Understand that the liver is the organ responsible for strategy… know that the Ancient Chinese called the Liver meridian the chief of staff, the official that makes vital strategy within the holistic system of organs throughout the body ...... while the gall bladder decides and discerns, liver plans and strategizes ... The power of the liver is strategy and vitality ....

Allow yourself to see that your key to achieving your dreams and desires lies in your understanding that you are the keeper of your vitality and essence… you are also responsible for your authentic voice, the key to knowing yourself and what you want and why, which in turn has the capacity to deliver the best you…

Become aware of the fact that you cannot control the outer world, understand that control of the outer world is an illusion ... and better understanding your meridians positions you to gain far greater control of your inner world…

Know that holding on to anger, fear, depression and baggage that no longer serves you will stagnate your liver Qi ... know that overworking yourself will rob you of your vitality… let go… relax… focus on kindness and breathe vitality and essence into your liver meridian…

Visualize one thing that you have been carrying around for too long… one burden that it is now time to let go of… see yourself setting it down… and now, see yourself walking away from it… longer weighing you down… feel how light you feel… feel your vitality surge…

Embrace the fact that over the course of 2,500 years, Traditional Chinese Medicine has become a tried and tested system of rational medicine known for its great diversity of healing and wellness practices ... know that the main goal of TCM is to create harmony between our mind, body, and the environment around us...

Understand that one very important way to create harmony is by making sure your Qi is balanced ... Qi means life energy and it stands for the energy in all things...

Your Qi provides the energy for important bodily functions like your digestion, metabolism, and overall strength ... It is also represented in other physical aspects of energy like sunlight, and electricity ... But other aspects like your thoughts and emotions are also powered by your Qi....

Let your mind drift to the magic of the meridians and how they work like a network system, transporting and distributing Qi and blood ... how the meridians link up organs, limbs, joints, bones, tendons, tissues and skin, and provide communication between the body interior and exterior, through a healthy meridian system...

Marvel at the magic of how Qi and blood successfully warm and nourish different organs and tissues, and maintain normal metabolic activities...

Understand that meridians are essential in supporting the flow of nutritive Qi inside the blood vessels and flow of protective Qi around them ... they strengthen the body's immunity, protect against external pernicious influences and assist in regulating Yin and Yang ...

Your Qi can become unbalanced due to a lack of nutritious food, clean, mineralized water, good sleep, and fresh air ... By nourishing your body and staying in harmony with your environment, you'll be able to restore and balance your Qi ... nutritious food... restorative sleep... herbal teas... time spent in nature... and of course meditation can all serve to balance your Qi... and so can deep breathing and of course acupuncture... be kind to yourself... engage in activities that that serve to balance your Qi...

Give yourself permission to embrace a new awareness of your power to create reality through the balancing your Qi and your meridians through meditation and how this awareness will prepare you to live unconditionally...

Understand that you must be careful when taking medicines as they affect the liver and the liver's detoxification role ... always remember that when lying down the blood belongs to the liver and it is important to close your eyes… it is also important to try to go to sleep when you go to bed and not ruminate, instead allowing the liver essence to detoxify the blood and replenish your vitality…

Know that the liver is about life and death, vitality and essence ... keep the liver in warmth… let go of what no longer serves you… stay away from anger, depression ... be kind to yourself and others

Notice the happiness you feel inside knowing how powerful meridian balance is and how connected to humanity you are…notice how this connection fills you with an elevated vibration… and how an elevated vibration can expand the visible spectrums of your senses…

Now just breathe and be with yourself and let the waves of your breathing be with you…

REVIEW

We have completed a pass through the 12 main meridians. Let's remember the order of the twelve meridians:

Arm: Lung Meridian to Large Intestine
Leg: Stomach Meridian to Spleen Meridian
Arm: Heart Meridian to Small Intestine
Leg: Bladder Meridian to Kidney Meridian
Arm: Pericardium Meridian to Triple Warmer
Leg: Gallbladder to Liver.

Flow of Qi - Although it is said that the circulation of the meridians is unprovoked, this sequence is indeed connected end to end.

For example, the lung meridian, which originates from the middle Jiao... straight out from the inner arm of the wrist, next to the inner finger, and out of the end, at the Shangyang Lung -1 point of the index finger.

It connects with the large intestine meridian; and the large intestine meridian starts from Lu-1 Shangyang and ends at large intestine 20 Yingxiang acupoint on both sides of the nostril, where it connects with the stomach meridian.

The stomach meridian starts from the nose and ends at the St-45 Lidui point of the second toe, and its branch enters the inner end of the big toe Sp-1 Yinbai acupoint and connects with the stomach meridian.

The stomach to the spleen meridian too is connected; the spleen meridian starts from SP-1 Yinbai point, and finally connects with the heart meridian;

The heart meridian starts from the heart and so it goes in this connected way, the lung meridian is connected to the large intestine meridian, the stomach meridian is connected to the spleen meridian, etc., that is, the internal and external connection of the Zang-Fu organs.

Once the principle of connection is understood, it is very convenient for us to learn Chinese medicine.

For example, the lungs and the large intestine are external and internal, the spleen and stomach are external and internal, the heart and the small intestine are external and internal, the bladder and the kidneys are external and internal, the pericardium and the triple warmer are external and internal, and the gallbladder and the liver are external and internal.

The heart is the official of the monarchy, and has the ability to control spirits. If the spirits are in chaos, the official of the monarch cannot control the whole body, the twelve officials will be in danger, and the whole body is not well. The official of the monarch is not concerned with specific matters, but is responsible for the stability of the spirits, with a leisurely mind and a leisurely body. So, take care of your spirits and your emotions first.

The lungs are the officials of the prime ministers, and the ability is to govern the energy and blood circulation, which should be balanced and controlled.

The liver is the official of the generals, and the ability is deliberation, which contains vitality.

The gallbladder is the official of justice, and the ability is the decision. If gallbladder has weak growth energy, then the bone is weak. To treat bone disease, we must first treat gallbladder growth.

The spleen, the official of the treasury/granary, and the ability is extracting the energy from food and beverages, and spreads the four directions. If the spleen meridian does not function properly, Qi cannot be efficiently transported to the spleen.

The stomach, minister of the mill, the five flavors come out, the main function is for receiving the food and beverage. If the stomach is sick and the stomach is insufficient then the Qi and blood will be insufficient.

The large intestine, the official of transportation. The ability is transformation. If the large intestine has weak transformation then its body fluids are self-injured.

The small intestine, the official of the minister of reception, possesses the ability of absorption. If the small intestine has weak absorption, then the nutrition is insufficient, and the immunity of the person is low.

The kidney, the official minister of power, from which the ability of ingenuity is derived. If the kidney is weak, it will cause decline of human creativity.

The bladder, the official of the minister of the reservoir, the ability to collect and store the body fluids, transform and distribute to the rest of the body. The main function is to control tendon's disease. If the bladder is strong, the tendons won't be sick.

The triple warmer is the official in charge of irrigation, the waterway. Triple warmer has the ability to control the Qi and meridian. If the triple warmer is weak, people's meridians will be sick.

The pericardium is the ambassador to the other officials from it joy and happiness derives. The main function is to regulate energy.

As a human being, you must first have the ability to store essence, learn and accumulate experience, and then you can know what you can do in the end, or where you are lacking, and what is wrong. At the same time, after collecting the essence of heaven and earth, you have to pay back according to your ability. Only by paying back can life be meaningful.

As far as the human body is concerned, it can basically be divided into three parts, the head, the cavity, and the limbs.

The Head: There are six meridians going to the head.

The first is the governor vessel. When the governor vessel enters the sea of marrow, it enters the brain.

The second one is the bladder meridian. The upper forehead crosses the top. It enters the brain from the top of the top. The bladder meridian is responsible for Yang Qi. Now many people have amnesia. In fact, amnesia is a disease of weak Yang Qi. The bladder meridian enters the brain, causing people to lose things and forget things.

Third, the liver meridian. "On the forehead, and the governor will meet at the top." In our human body, the three internal organs of the brain, heart, and kidney cannot be ischemia (restricted blood and therefore oxygen flow) at any moment. Liver blood deficiency, headache and insomnia.

Fourth, the stomach meridian "runs from the hairline to the forehead."

The nutrients we eat must be transported to the heart and lungs through the stomach meridian, and also to the brain.

The fifth, sixth, the Yang and Yin heel meridians in eight extraordinary meridians, all enter the back of the brain, and the back of the brain controls our motor coordination.

The most common encephalopathy are cerebral hemorrhage and cerebral thrombosis. People in their 50s and 60s may suffer from cerebral hemorrhage after big and intense stress or anger, the reason is whether the vitality is full. If the vitality is sufficient, the blood will not be sticky, and the peripheral blood vessels will be elastic and not brittle. This is also the reason why people in their twenties will not suffer from this disease even if they are angry.

Cerebral thrombosis is also the lack of vitality, unable to push the blood up to the brain, causing the blood to flow slowly or even stop, causing the blood to coagulate at the end of the blood vessels in the brain, forming a thrombus. Coupled with the cold autumn and winter, it is easy to fall ill. In mild cases, the fingertips are numb, and in severe cases, cerebral thrombosis will occur.

What nourishes the brain the most?

Sleep. During the day, Wei Qi travels in the Yang element of the human body, and at night it travels in the Yin element, that is, the Yin meridian. As long as the Yang Qi enters the Yin meridian, people want to sleep. After Wei Qi has done in the Yin meridian, the moment it leaves the Yin meridian, a person will wake up. Sleep is actually the embodiment of the regularity of the meridians.

Massage the scalp: use fingers or comb to massage or stimulate the scalp every day 100 times.

There are the five viscera and six Fu-organs, which can be divided into three sections. The twelve meridians are all distributed in the cavity. Here the emphasis is mainly on the upper and lower opening of the cavity.

The upper opening:

The throat, and there are as many as nine meridians that go through the throat. The large intestine meridian, the stomach meridian, the spleen meridian, the heart meridian, the small intestine meridian, the kidney meridian, the liver meridian, the du meridian and ren meridian.

All the meridians of the upper brain and the upper head must pass through the throat, so it can be seen that the throat is indeed a significant point, which can block the upward movement of the disease. How can the tonsils be operated on? Moreover, throat diseases are basically classified as all emotional diseases will first manifest in the throat, so throat diseases are relatively serious diseases.

How to take care throat and neck area:

Slowly rotate the neck in both directions 100 times every day, you might hear cracking sounds in the beginning, as you do more, the sounds will diminish.

Scrap the neck and throat area with a jade scraper until the skin turns red.

Wear a scarf on windy and cold days.

Manage your emotions.

Openings in the lower cavity: Genitals, urinary track and anus.

The main meridians that run through the genitals are: ren, chong, du, liver, gallbladder; kidney and bladder meridians also go to the anus and buttocks.

Ren, Du, Chong meridians are extraordinary meridians which we have not covered in this program. The Ren meridian, which originates from the uterus, and after it comes out of the perineum of the human body, it directly rushes upward from the bottom and runs in the middle of the front of the body; the second is the Chong Meridian, which also comes out from the perineum and rushes from the bottom to the top, runs inside of middle of body. It is the process of human sexual development, a key meridian in the middle. Then the Du meridian, which originates from the lower abdomen, enters the vagina for women, and descends from the penis for men, then rise up in the spine up to head.

What are men most afraid of? Impotence and premature ejaculation. People with these conditions often have violent tendencies in order to cover up their perceived deficiency.

There are basically four causes of impotence:

Liver blood deficiency, kidney Yang deficiency, kidney Yin deficiency, and bladder meridian Qi deficiency. Young people are basically related to excessive masturbation, and middle-aged people are related to excessive stress. Diabetic patients suffer from impotence syndrome, which means that they belong to the syndrome of Yang deficiency. At this time, impotence is a self-protection function.

If the husband has the problem of impotence and premature ejaculation, most of the wives will suffer from hormone imbalance, or other gynecological inflammations, and the severe ones will suffer from uterine fibroids. Because the uterus can stagnate, it needs the stimulation and agitation of Yang Qi. People who have not been able to have sexual pleasure for a long time are like flowers that have never bloomed. A small amount of mucus secreted by emotion accumulates in the vaginal wall and cannot be discharged in time. It will accumulate and condense into leucorrhea, which will turn yellow and stinky over time. Coupled with depression and fatigue, it will cause gynecological inflammation. In other words, if the fertile fields cannot get good seeds, weeds will grow, cysts and fibroids will grow.

The pathology of female diseases is the same as that of men's nocturnal emission, impotence and premature ejaculation, so the treatment methods are basically the same.

How to protect Kidneys:

A few ways to protect the kidney were discussed in the kidney meridian chapter, and here we will add two more points.

First, when you go to the bathroom, you cannot speak. Grit your teeth, because the teeth are associated with the kidneys, the manifestation of the essence of the kidneys. Men should lift the heels.

The second is that when you sit, the two hands are firmly grasped, or sit with two legs crossed, like a lock, locking the lower burner, so that people will calm down, and the Qi will run in ren and du meridians.

Limbs

The most important part of the limbs is the joints.

The heart meridian and the lung meridian go through the shoulder joint, elbow joint and wrist joint, the large intestine meridian is upper shoulder. The stomach meridian goes through the hip and knee joints.

The spleen meridian passes pelvic bone, inside of leg and inner ankle.

The small intestine passes around the scapula and over the shoulder, as well as the wrist.

The bladder goes to the lower back,

The kidney meridian goes to the heel and so on.

How to Protect Limbs:

Keep warm: For the human body, the cervical spine and throat are the most vulnerable at the top, the waist is the most vulnerable in the middle, and the ankles are the most vulnerable at the bottom, so the ankles also need to be protected. It needs to be emphasized that the cervical spine, the waist, navel, and the ankles should not be exposed to cold. These three key points of the human body are all pivotal places, and none of them can suffer from cold. Once cold, it will cause a series of diseases.

Soaking your feet has almost unlimited benefits. When soaking your feet, they must be soaked to above the ankle. Even better to soak up to the calf! This is a very important health care principle.

Exercise.

Foot

The meridians of the feet are from the inside to the outside: the spleen, liver, stomach, gallbladder and bladder.

The spleen meridian enters the big toe, going through Yinbai SP-1 point.

The liver meridian also enters the big toe Liver -1 Dadun point.

The stomach meridian goes to the second toe, but it divides into three branches, one enters the inner side of the second toe, and then goes through the ST-44 Nei Ting point; one enters the outside of the middle toe; one ends at the end of the big toe SP-1 Yinbai point, connected to the spleen meridian. The stomach and spleen communication between yin and yang is at Yinbai acupoint.

The gallbladder meridian goes to the posterior lateral side of the fourth toe of the foot, GB 44 Qiaoyin point.

The bladder meridian goes to the UB 67 Zhi Yin point outside the little toe.

Because the hands move every day, the feet move less, and they are far away from the viscera, so the maintenance of the feet is very important.

SP-1 Yinbai, Kid - 1 Yongquan, Liver 3 Taichong all specialize in the treatment of mental patients, so soaking feet can at least calm the mind, but it is better if you can rub your toes vigorously.

The heart controls the blood vessels, if the feet are warm, the heart and lung function will be normal. If the toes are cold, the points of the spleen, liver, bladder, stomach, and gallbladder on toes will all be blocked, and people will feel uncomfortable.

There are two indicators for a person to be seriously ill. One is that he can't sleep all night, and the other is that his legs and feet are getting cold and freezing. These are indicators that a person is seriously ill.

From studying the meridians, you can establish a correct way of thinking, and use Qi, Yin and Yang, and the five elements to see the world, not only from one more unique angle, but also from an angle that has the capacity to create pleasure.

Second, there are many ways to maintain health. Most of us were not taught that keeping our mind quiet is good for our health. Now we understand that the spirits, Yang, etc., go through the seven orifices. The important way to calm your mind and spirits is to be mindful of what you expose yourself to, see and hear less chaotic things.

Third, love yourself and all beings better. We must not think that only medicine can cure disease, our language can also cure disease, and our mentality can also cure disease. When our body and mind are softened, the world will reward us with tenderness.

We have reached the end of the meditation with meridians presentation. Once again, the biggest medicine is in our body, the meridians! The best doctor is ourselves! Hope you all stay in good health!

Thank you all for following along and we hope you have enjoyed learning about the meridians and joining knowledge of the meridians with meditation!